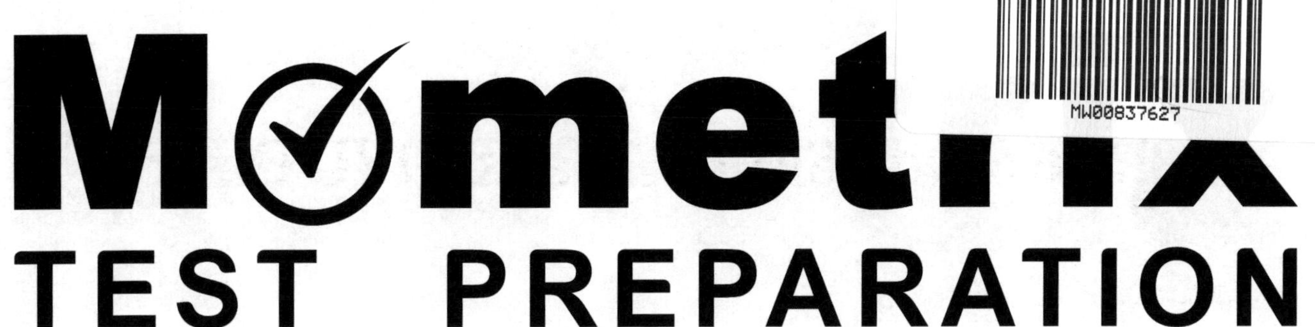

Vascular Sonography Exam Secrets Study Guide

Dear Future Exam Success Story

First of all, **THANK YOU** for purchasing Mometrix study materials!

Second, congratulations! You are one of the few determined test-takers who are committed to doing whatever it takes to excel on your exam. **You have come to the right place.** We developed these study materials with one goal in mind: to deliver you the information you need in a format that's concise and easy to use.

In addition to optimizing your guide for the content of the test, we've outlined our recommended steps for breaking down the preparation process into small, attainable goals so you can make sure you stay on track.

We've also analyzed the entire test-taking process, identifying the most common pitfalls and showing how you can overcome them and be ready for any curveball the test throws you.

Standardized testing is one of the biggest obstacles on your road to success, which only increases the importance of doing well in the high-pressure, high-stakes environment of test day. Your results on this test could have a significant impact on your future, and this guide provides the information and practical advice to help you achieve your full potential on test day.

Your success is our success

We would love to hear from you! If you would like to share the story of your exam success or if you have any questions or comments in regard to our products, please contact us at **800-673-8175** or **support@mometrix.com**.

Thanks again for your business and we wish you continued success!

Sincerely,
The Mometrix Test Preparation Team

Need more help? Check out our flashcards at:
http://mometrixflashcards.com/ARRT

Copyright © 2022 by Mometrix Media LLC. All rights reserved.
Written and edited by the Mometrix Exam Secrets Test Prep Team
Printed in the United States of America

Table of Contents

Introduction

Thank you for purchasing this resource! You have made the choice to prepare yourself for a test that could have a huge impact on your future, and this guide is designed to help you be fully ready for test day. Obviously, it's important to have a solid understanding of the test material, but you also need to be prepared for the unique environment and stressors of the test, so that you can perform to the best of your abilities.

For this purpose, the first section that appears in this guide is the **Secret Keys**. We've devoted countless hours to meticulously researching what works and what doesn't, and we've boiled down our findings to the five most impactful steps you can take to improve your performance on the test. We start at the beginning with study planning and move through the preparation process, all the way to the testing strategies that will help you get the most out of what you know when you're finally sitting in front of the test.

We recommend that you start preparing for your test as far in advance as possible. However, if you've bought this guide as a last-minute study resource and only have a few days before your test, we recommend that you skip over the first two Secret Keys since they address a long-term study plan.

If you struggle with **test anxiety**, we strongly encourage you to check out our recommendations for how you can overcome it. Test anxiety is a formidable foe, but it can be beaten, and we want to make sure you have the tools you need to defeat it.

Copyright © Mometrix Media. You have been licensed one copy of this document for personal use only. Any other reproduction or redistribution is strictly prohibited. All rights reserved.
This content is provided for test preparation purposes only and does not imply an endorsement by Mometrix of any particular political, scientific, or religious point of view.

Secret Key #1 – Plan Big, Study Small

There's a lot riding on your performance. If you want to ace this test, you're going to need to keep your skills sharp and the material fresh in your mind. You need a plan that lets you review everything you need to know while still fitting in your schedule. We'll break this strategy down into three categories.

Information Organization

Start with the information you already have: the official test outline. From this, you can make a complete list of all the concepts you need to cover before the test. Organize these concepts into groups that can be studied together, and create a list of any related vocabulary you need to learn so you can brush up on any difficult terms. You'll want to keep this vocabulary list handy once you actually start studying since you may need to add to it along the way.

Time Management

Once you have your set of study concepts, decide how to spread them out over the time you have left before the test. Break your study plan into small, clear goals so you have a manageable task for each day and know exactly what you're doing. Then just focus on one small step at a time. When you manage your time this way, you don't need to spend hours at a time studying. Studying a small block of content for a short period each day helps you retain information better and avoid stressing over how much you have left to do. You can relax knowing that you have a plan to cover everything in time. In order for this strategy to be effective though, you have to start studying early and stick to your schedule. Avoid the exhaustion and futility that comes from last-minute cramming!

Study Environment

The environment you study in has a big impact on your learning. Studying in a coffee shop, while probably more enjoyable, is not likely to be as fruitful as studying in a quiet room. It's important to keep distractions to a minimum. You're only planning to study for a short block of time, so make the most of it. Don't pause to check your phone or get up to find a snack. It's also important to **avoid multitasking**. Research has consistently shown that multitasking will make your studying dramatically less effective. Your study area should also be comfortable and well-lit so you don't have the distraction of straining your eyes or sitting on an uncomfortable chair.

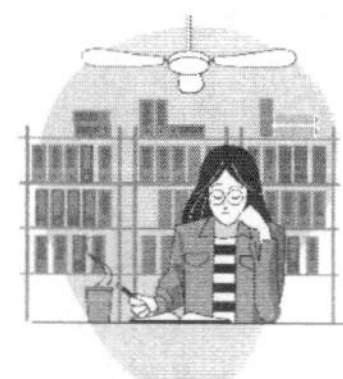

The time of day you study is also important. You want to be rested and alert. Don't wait until just before bedtime. Study when you'll be most likely to comprehend and remember. Even better, if you know what time of day your test will be, set that time aside for study. That way your brain will be used to working on that subject at that specific time and you'll have a better chance of recalling information.

Finally, it can be helpful to team up with others who are studying for the same test. Your actual studying should be done in as isolated an environment as possible, but the work of organizing the information and setting up the study plan can be divided up. In between study sessions, you can discuss with your teammates the concepts that you're all studying and quiz each other on the details. Just be sure that your teammates are as serious about the test as you are. If you find that your study time is being replaced with social time, you might need to find a new team.

Copyright © Mometrix Media. You have been licensed one copy of this document for personal use only. Any other reproduction or redistribution is strictly prohibited. All rights reserved.
This content is provided for test preparation purposes only and does not imply an endorsement by Mometrix of any particular political, scientific, or religious point of view.

Secret Key #2 – Make Your Studying Count

You're devoting a lot of time and effort to preparing for this test, so you want to be absolutely certain it will pay off. This means doing more than just reading the content and hoping you can remember it on test day. It's important to make every minute of study count. There are two main areas you can focus on to make your studying count.

Retention

It doesn't matter how much time you study if you can't remember the material. You need to make sure you are retaining the concepts. To check your retention of the information you're learning, try recalling it at later times with minimal prompting. Try carrying around flashcards and glance at one or two from time to time or ask a friend who's also studying for the test to quiz you.

To enhance your retention, look for ways to put the information into practice so that you can apply it rather than simply recalling it. If you're using the information in practical ways, it will be much easier to remember. Similarly, it helps to solidify a concept in your mind if you're not only reading it to yourself but also explaining it to someone else. Ask a friend to let you teach them about a concept you're a little shaky on (or speak aloud to an imaginary audience if necessary). As you try to summarize, define, give examples, and answer your friend's questions, you'll understand the concepts better and they will stay with you longer. Finally, step back for a big picture view and ask yourself how each piece of information fits with the whole subject. When you link the different concepts together and see them working together as a whole, it's easier to remember the individual components.

Finally, practice showing your work on any multi-step problems, even if you're just studying. Writing out each step you take to solve a problem will help solidify the process in your mind, and you'll be more likely to remember it during the test.

Modality

Modality simply refers to the means or method by which you study. Choosing a study modality that fits your own individual learning style is crucial. No two people learn best in exactly the same way, so it's important to know your strengths and use them to your advantage.

For example, if you learn best by visualization, focus on visualizing a concept in your mind and draw an image or a diagram. Try color-coding your notes, illustrating them, or creating symbols that will trigger your mind to recall a learned concept. If you learn best by hearing or discussing information, find a study partner who learns the same way or read aloud to yourself. Think about how to put the information in your own words. Imagine that you are giving a lecture on the topic and record yourself so you can listen to it later.

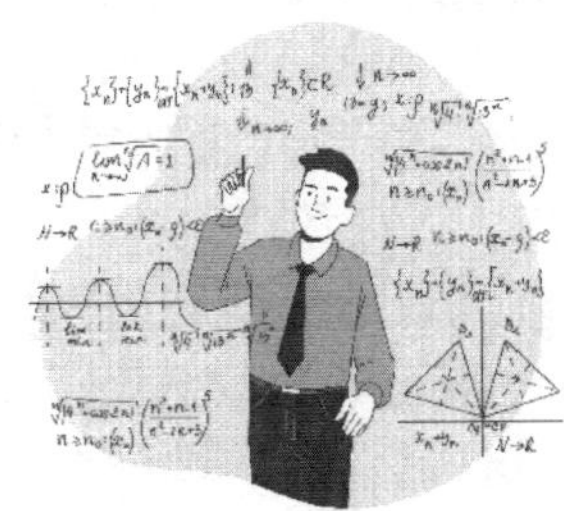

For any learning style, flashcards can be helpful. Organize the information so you can take advantage of spare moments to review. Underline key words or phrases. Use different colors for different categories. Mnemonic devices (such as creating a short list in which every item starts with the same letter) can also help with retention. Find what works best for you and use it to store the information in your mind most effectively and easily.

Copyright © Mometrix Media. You have been licensed one copy of this document for personal use only. Any other reproduction or redistribution is strictly prohibited. All rights reserved.
This content is provided for test preparation purposes only and does not imply an endorsement by Mometrix of any particular political, scientific, or religious point of view.

Secret Key #3 – Practice the Right Way

Your success on test day depends not only on how many hours you put into preparing, but also on whether you prepared the right way. It's good to check along the way to see if your studying is paying off. One of the most effective ways to do this is by taking practice tests to evaluate your progress. Practice tests are useful because they show exactly where you need to improve. Every time you take a practice test, pay special attention to these three groups of questions:

- The questions you got wrong
- The questions you had to guess on, even if you guessed right
- The questions you found difficult or slow to work through

This will show you exactly what your weak areas are, and where you need to devote more study time. Ask yourself why each of these questions gave you trouble. Was it because you didn't understand the material? Was it because you didn't remember the vocabulary? Do you need more repetitions on this type of question to build speed and confidence? Dig into those questions and figure out how you can strengthen your weak areas as you go back to review the material.

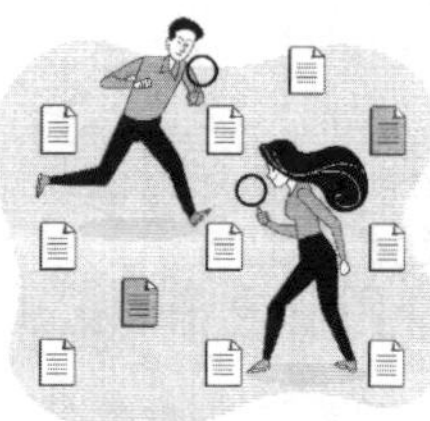

Additionally, many practice tests have a section explaining the answer choices. It can be tempting to read the explanation and think that you now have a good understanding of the concept. However, an explanation likely only covers part of the question's broader context. Even if the explanation makes perfect sense, **go back and investigate** every concept related to the question until you're positive you have a thorough understanding.

As you go along, keep in mind that the practice test is just that: practice. Memorizing these questions and answers will not be very helpful on the actual test because it is unlikely to have any of the same exact questions. If you only know the right answers to the sample questions, you won't be prepared for the real thing. **Study the concepts** until you understand them fully, and then you'll be able to answer any question that shows up on the test.

It's important to wait on the practice tests until you're ready. If you take a test on your first day of study, you may be overwhelmed by the amount of material covered and how much you need to learn. Work up to it gradually.

On test day, you'll need to be prepared for answering questions, managing your time, and using the test-taking strategies you've learned. It's a lot to balance, like a mental marathon that will have a big impact on your future. Like training for a marathon, you'll need to start slowly and work your way up. When test day arrives, you'll be ready.

Start with the strategies you've read in the first two Secret Keys—plan your course and study in the way that works best for you. If you have time, consider using multiple study resources to get different approaches to the same concepts. It can be helpful to see difficult concepts from more than one angle. Then find a good source for practice tests. Many times, the test website will suggest potential study resources or provide sample tests.

Copyright © Mometrix Media. You have been licensed one copy of this document for personal use only. Any other reproduction or redistribution is strictly prohibited. All rights reserved.
This content is provided for test preparation purposes only and does not imply an endorsement by Mometrix of any particular political, scientific, or religious point of view.

Practice Test Strategy

If you're able to find at least three practice tests, we recommend this strategy:

Untimed and Open-Book Practice

Take the first test with no time constraints and with your notes and study guide handy. Take your time and focus on applying the strategies you've learned.

Timed and Open-Book Practice

Take the second practice test open-book as well, but set a timer and practice pacing yourself to finish in time.

Timed and Closed-Book Practice

Take any other practice tests as if it were test day. Set a timer and put away your study materials. Sit at a table or desk in a quiet room, imagine yourself at the testing center, and answer questions as quickly and accurately as possible.

Keep repeating timed and closed-book tests on a regular basis until you run out of practice tests or it's time for the actual test. Your mind will be ready for the schedule and stress of test day, and you'll be able to focus on recalling the material you've learned.

Copyright © Mometrix Media. You have been licensed one copy of this document for personal use only. Any other reproduction or redistribution is strictly prohibited. All rights reserved.
This content is provided for test preparation purposes only and does not imply an endorsement by Mometrix of any particular political, scientific, or religious point of view.

Secret Key #4 – Pace Yourself

Once you're fully prepared for the material on the test, your biggest challenge on test day will be managing your time. Just knowing that the clock is ticking can make you panic even if you have plenty of time left. Work on pacing yourself so you can build confidence against the time constraints of the exam. Pacing is a difficult skill to master, especially in a high-pressure environment, so **practice is vital**.

Set time expectations for your pace based on how much time is available. For example, if a section has 60 questions and the time limit is 30 minutes, you know you have to average 30 seconds or less per question in order to answer them all. Although 30 seconds is the hard limit, set 25 seconds per question as your goal, so you reserve extra time to spend on harder questions. When you budget extra time for the harder questions, you no longer have any reason to stress when those questions take longer to answer.

Don't let this time expectation distract you from working through the test at a calm, steady pace, but keep it in mind so you don't spend too much time on any one question. Recognize that taking extra time on one question you don't understand may keep you from answering two that you do understand later in the test. If your time limit for a question is up and you're still not sure of the answer, mark it and move on, and come back to it later if the time and the test format allow. If the testing format doesn't allow you to return to earlier questions, just make an educated guess; then put it out of your mind and move on.

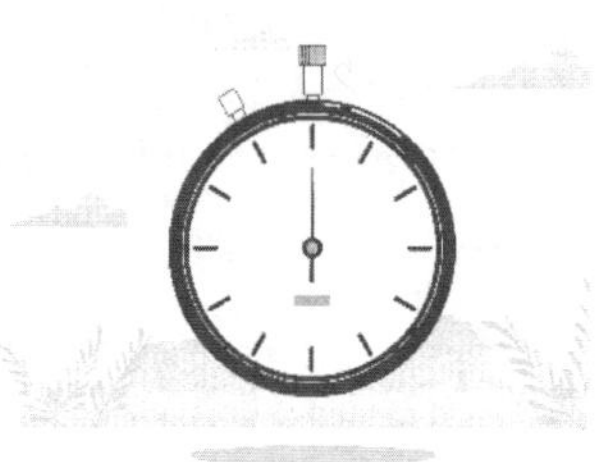

On the easier questions, be careful not to rush. It may seem wise to hurry through them so you have more time for the challenging ones, but it's not worth missing one if you know the concept and just didn't take the time to read the question fully. Work efficiently but make sure you understand the question and have looked at all of the answer choices, since more than one may seem right at first.

Even if you're paying attention to the time, you may find yourself a little behind at some point. You should speed up to get back on track, but do so wisely. Don't panic; just take a few seconds less on each question until you're caught up. Don't guess without thinking, but do look through the answer choices and eliminate any you know are wrong. If you can get down to two choices, it is often worthwhile to guess from those. Once you've chosen an answer, move on and don't dwell on any that you skipped or had to hurry through. If a question was taking too long, chances are it was one of the harder ones, so you weren't as likely to get it right anyway.

On the other hand, if you find yourself getting ahead of schedule, it may be beneficial to slow down a little. The more quickly you work, the more likely you are to make a careless mistake that will affect your score. You've budgeted time for each question, so don't be afraid to spend that time. Practice an efficient but careful pace to get the most out of the time you have.

Copyright © Mometrix Media. You have been licensed one copy of this document for personal use only. Any other reproduction or redistribution is strictly prohibited. All rights reserved.
This content is provided for test preparation purposes only and does not imply an endorsement by Mometrix of any particular political, scientific, or religious point of view.

Secret Key #5 – Have a Plan for Guessing

When you're taking the test, you may find yourself stuck on a question. Some of the answer choices seem better than others, but you don't see the one answer choice that is obviously correct. What do you do?

The scenario described above is very common, yet most test takers have not effectively prepared for it. Developing and practicing a plan for guessing may be one of the single most effective uses of your time as you get ready for the exam.

In developing your plan for guessing, there are three questions to address:

- When should you start the guessing process?
- How should you narrow down the choices?
- Which answer should you choose?

When to Start the Guessing Process

Unless your plan for guessing is to select C every time (which, despite its merits, is not what we recommend), you need to leave yourself enough time to apply your answer elimination strategies. Since you have a limited amount of time for each question, that means that if you're going to give yourself the best shot at guessing correctly, you have to decide quickly whether or not you will guess.

Of course, the best-case scenario is that you don't have to guess at all, so first, see if you can answer the question based on your knowledge of the subject and basic reasoning skills. Focus on the key words in the question and try to jog your memory of related topics. Give yourself a chance to bring the knowledge to mind, but once you realize that you don't have (or you can't access) the knowledge you need to answer the question, it's time to start the guessing process.

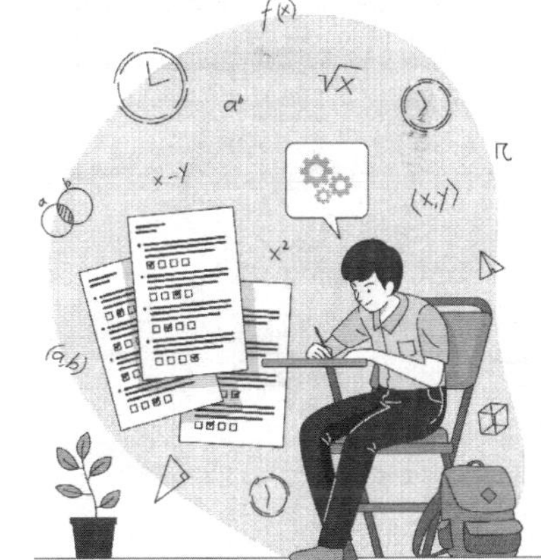

It's almost always better to start the guessing process too early than too late. It only takes a few seconds to remember something and answer the question from knowledge. Carefully eliminating wrong answer choices takes longer. Plus, going through the process of eliminating answer choices can actually help jog your memory.

Summary: Start the guessing process as soon as you decide that you can't answer the question based on your knowledge.

Copyright © Mometrix Media. You have been licensed one copy of this document for personal use only. Any other reproduction or redistribution is strictly prohibited. All rights reserved.
This content is provided for test preparation purposes only and does not imply an endorsement by Mometrix of any particular political, scientific, or religious point of view.

How to Narrow Down the Choices

The next chapter in this book (**Test-Taking Strategies**) includes a wide range of strategies for how to approach questions and how to look for answer choices to eliminate. You will definitely want to read those carefully, practice them, and figure out which ones work best for you. Here though, we're going to address a mindset rather than a particular strategy.

Your odds of guessing an answer correctly depend on how many options you are choosing from.

Number of options left	5	4	3	2	1
Odds of guessing correctly	20%	25%	33%	50%	100%

You can see from this chart just how valuable it is to be able to eliminate incorrect answers and make an educated guess, but there are two things that many test takers do that cause them to miss out on the benefits of guessing:

- Accidentally eliminating the correct answer
- Selecting an answer based on an impression

We'll look at the first one here, and the second one in the next section.

To avoid accidentally eliminating the correct answer, we recommend a thought exercise called **the $5 challenge**. In this challenge, you only eliminate an answer choice from contention if you are willing to bet $5 on it being wrong. Why $5? Five dollars is a small but not insignificant amount of money. It's an amount you could afford to lose but wouldn't want to throw away. And while losing $5 once might not hurt too much, doing it twenty times will set you back $100. In the same way, each small decision you make—eliminating a choice here, guessing on a question there—won't by itself impact your score very much, but when you put them all together, they can make a big difference. By holding each answer choice elimination decision to a higher standard, you can reduce the risk of accidentally eliminating the correct answer.

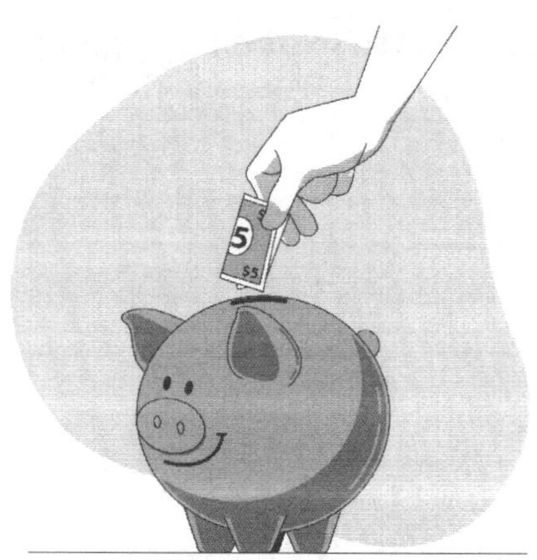

The $5 challenge can also be applied in a positive sense: If you are willing to bet $5 that an answer choice *is* correct, go ahead and mark it as correct.

Summary: Only eliminate an answer choice if you are willing to bet $5 that it is wrong.

Copyright © Mometrix Media. You have been licensed one copy of this document for personal use only. Any other reproduction or redistribution is strictly prohibited. All rights reserved.
This content is provided for test preparation purposes only and does not imply an endorsement by Mometrix of any particular political, scientific, or religious point of view.

Which Answer to Choose

You're taking the test. You've run into a hard question and decided you'll have to guess. You've eliminated all the answer choices you're willing to bet $5 on. Now you have to pick an answer. Why do we even need to talk about this? Why can't you just pick whichever one you feel like when the time comes?

The answer to these questions is that if you don't come into the test with a plan, you'll rely on your impression to select an answer choice, and if you do that, you risk falling into a trap. The test writers know that everyone who takes their test will be guessing on some of the questions, so they intentionally write wrong answer choices to seem plausible. You still have to pick an answer though, and if the wrong answer choices are designed to look right, how can you ever be sure that you're not falling for their trap? The best solution we've found to this dilemma is to take the decision out of your hands entirely. Here is the process we recommend:

Once you've eliminated any choices that you are confident (willing to bet $5) are wrong, select the first remaining choice as your answer.

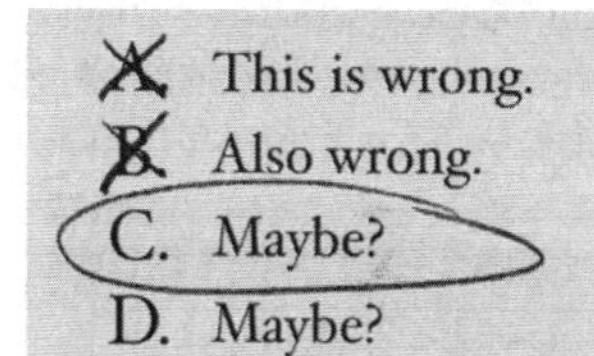

Whether you choose to select the first remaining choice, the second, or the last, the important thing is that you use some preselected standard. Using this approach guarantees that you will not be enticed into selecting an answer choice that looks right, because you are not basing your decision on how the answer choices look.

This is not meant to make you question your knowledge. Instead, it is to help you recognize the difference between your knowledge and your impressions. There's a huge difference between thinking an answer is right because of what you know, and thinking an answer is right because it looks or sounds like it should be right.

Summary: To ensure that your selection is appropriately random, make a predetermined selection from among all answer choices you have not eliminated.

Copyright © Mometrix Media. You have been licensed one copy of this document for personal use only. Any other reproduction or redistribution is strictly prohibited. All rights reserved.
This content is provided for test preparation purposes only and does not imply an endorsement by Mometrix of any particular political, scientific, or religious point of view.

Test-Taking Strategies

This section contains a list of test-taking strategies that you may find helpful as you work through the test. By taking what you know and applying logical thought, you can maximize your chances of answering any question correctly!

It is very important to realize that every question is different and every person is different: no single strategy will work on every question, and no single strategy will work for every person. That's why we've included all of them here, so you can try them out and determine which ones work best for different types of questions and which ones work best for you.

Question Strategies

✓ Read Carefully

Read the question and the answer choices carefully. Don't miss the question because you misread the terms. You have plenty of time to read each question thoroughly and make sure you understand what is being asked. Yet a happy medium must be attained, so don't waste too much time. You must read carefully and efficiently.

✓ Contextual Clues

Look for contextual clues. If the question includes a word you are not familiar with, look at the immediate context for some indication of what the word might mean. Contextual clues can often give you all the information you need to decipher the meaning of an unfamiliar word. Even if you can't determine the meaning, you may be able to narrow down the possibilities enough to make a solid guess at the answer to the question.

✓ Prefixes

If you're having trouble with a word in the question or answer choices, try dissecting it. Take advantage of every clue that the word might include. Prefixes can be a huge help. Usually, they allow you to determine a basic meaning. *Pre-* means before, *post-* means after, *pro-* is positive, *de-* is negative. From prefixes, you can get an idea of the general meaning of the word and try to put it into context.

✓ Hedge Words

Watch out for critical hedge words, such as *likely, may, can, sometimes, often, almost, mostly, usually, generally, rarely,* and *sometimes.* Question writers insert these hedge phrases to cover every possibility. Often an answer choice will be wrong simply because it leaves no room for exception. Be on guard for answer choices that have definitive words such as *exactly* and *always.*

✓ Switchback Words

Stay alert for *switchbacks.* These are the words and phrases frequently used to alert you to shifts in thought. The most common switchback words are *but, although,* and *however.* Others include *nevertheless, on the other hand, even though, while, in spite of, despite,* and *regardless of.* Switchback words are important to catch because they can change the direction of the question or an answer choice.

Copyright © Mometrix Media. You have been licensed one copy of this document for personal use only. Any other reproduction or redistribution is strictly prohibited. All rights reserved.
This content is provided for test preparation purposes only and does not imply an endorsement by Mometrix of any particular political, scientific, or religious point of view.

✓ Face Value

When in doubt, use common sense. Accept the situation in the problem at face value. Don't read too much into it. These problems will not require you to make wild assumptions. If you have to go beyond creativity and warp time or space in order to have an answer choice fit the question, then you should move on and consider the other answer choices. These are normal problems rooted in reality. The applicable relationship or explanation may not be readily apparent, but it is there for you to figure out. Use your common sense to interpret anything that isn't clear.

Answer Choice Strategies

✓ Answer Selection

The most thorough way to pick an answer choice is to identify and eliminate wrong answers until only one is left, then confirm it is the correct answer. Sometimes an answer choice may immediately seem right, but be careful. The test writers will usually put more than one reasonable answer choice on each question, so take a second to read all of them and make sure that the other choices are not equally obvious. As long as you have time left, it is better to read every answer choice than to pick the first one that looks right without checking the others.

✓ Answer Choice Families

An answer choice family consists of two (in rare cases, three) answer choices that are very similar in construction and cannot all be true at the same time. If you see two answer choices that are direct opposites or parallels, one of them is usually the correct answer. For instance, if one answer choice says that quantity *x* increases and another either says that quantity *x* decreases (opposite) or says that quantity *y* increases (parallel), then those answer choices would fall into the same family. An answer choice that doesn't match the construction of the answer choice family is more likely to be incorrect. Most questions will not have answer choice families, but when they do appear, you should be prepared to recognize them.

✓ Eliminate Answers

Eliminate answer choices as soon as you realize they are wrong, but make sure you consider all possibilities. If you are eliminating answer choices and realize that the last one you are left with is also wrong, don't panic. Start over and consider each choice again. There may be something you missed the first time that you will realize on the second pass.

✓ Avoid Fact Traps

Don't be distracted by an answer choice that is factually true but doesn't answer the question. You are looking for the choice that answers the question. Stay focused on what the question is asking for so you don't accidentally pick an answer that is true but incorrect. Always go back to the question and make sure the answer choice you've selected actually answers the question and is not merely a true statement.

✓ Extreme Statements

In general, you should avoid answers that put forth extreme actions as standard practice or proclaim controversial ideas as established fact. An answer choice that states the "process should be used in certain situations, if..." is much more likely to be correct than one that states the "process should be discontinued completely." The first is a calm rational statement and doesn't even make a definitive, uncompromising stance, using a hedge word *if* to provide wiggle room, whereas the second choice is far more extreme.

Copyright © Mometrix Media. You have been licensed one copy of this document for personal use only. Any other reproduction or redistribution is strictly prohibited. All rights reserved.
This content is provided for test preparation purposes only and does not imply an endorsement by Mometrix of any particular political, scientific, or religious point of view.

⊘ Benchmark

As you read through the answer choices and you come across one that seems to answer the question well, mentally select that answer choice. This is not your final answer, but it's the one that will help you evaluate the other answer choices. The one that you selected is your benchmark or standard for judging each of the other answer choices. Every other answer choice must be compared to your benchmark. That choice is correct until proven otherwise by another answer choice beating it. If you find a better answer, then that one becomes your new benchmark. Once you've decided that no other choice answers the question as well as your benchmark, you have your final answer.

⊘ Predict the Answer

Before you even start looking at the answer choices, it is often best to try to predict the answer. When you come up with the answer on your own, it is easier to avoid distractions and traps because you will know exactly what to look for. The right answer choice is unlikely to be word-for-word what you came up with, but it should be a close match. Even if you are confident that you have the right answer, you should still take the time to read each option before moving on.

General Strategies

⊘ Tough Questions

If you are stumped on a problem or it appears too hard or too difficult, don't waste time. Move on! Remember though, if you can quickly check for obviously incorrect answer choices, your chances of guessing correctly are greatly improved. Before you completely give up, at least try to knock out a couple of possible answers. Eliminate what you can and then guess at the remaining answer choices before moving on.

⊘ Check Your Work

Since you will probably not know every term listed and the answer to every question, it is important that you get credit for the ones that you do know. Don't miss any questions through careless mistakes. If at all possible, try to take a second to look back over your answer selection and make sure you've selected the correct answer choice and haven't made a costly careless mistake (such as marking an answer choice that you didn't mean to mark). This quick double check should more than pay for itself in caught mistakes for the time it costs.

⊘ Pace Yourself

It's easy to be overwhelmed when you're looking at a page full of questions; your mind is confused and full of random thoughts, and the clock is ticking down faster than you would like. Calm down and maintain the pace that you have set for yourself. Especially as you get down to the last few minutes of the test, don't let the small numbers on the clock make you panic. As long as you are on track by monitoring your pace, you are guaranteed to have time for each question.

⊘ Don't Rush

It is very easy to make errors when you are in a hurry. Maintaining a fast pace in answering questions is pointless if it makes you miss questions that you would have gotten right otherwise. Test writers like to include distracting information and wrong answers that seem right. Taking a little extra time to avoid careless mistakes can make all the difference in your test score. Find a pace that allows you to be confident in the answers that you select.

Copyright © Mometrix Media. You have been licensed one copy of this document for personal use only. Any other reproduction or redistribution is strictly prohibited. All rights reserved.
This content is provided for test preparation purposes only and does not imply an endorsement by Mometrix of any particular political, scientific, or religious point of view.

⊘ Keep Moving

Panicking will not help you pass the test, so do your best to stay calm and keep moving. Taking deep breaths and going through the answer elimination steps you practiced can help to break through a stress barrier and keep your pace.

Final Notes

The combination of a solid foundation of content knowledge and the confidence that comes from practicing your plan for applying that knowledge is the key to maximizing your performance on test day. As your foundation of content knowledge is built up and strengthened, you'll find that the strategies included in this chapter become more and more effective in helping you quickly sift through the distractions and traps of the test to isolate the correct answer.

Now that you're preparing to move forward into the test content chapters of this book, be sure to keep your goal in mind. As you read, think about how you will be able to apply this information on the test. If you've already seen sample questions for the test and you have an idea of the question format and style, try to come up with questions of your own that you can answer based on what you're reading. This will give you valuable practice applying your knowledge in the same ways you can expect to on test day.

Good luck and good studying!

Copyright © Mometrix Media. You have been licensed one copy of this document for personal use only. Any other reproduction or redistribution is strictly prohibited. All rights reserved.
This content is provided for test preparation purposes only and does not imply an endorsement by Mometrix of any particular political, scientific, or religious point of view.

Copyright © Mometrix Media. You have been licensed one copy of this document for personal use only. Any other reproduction or redistribution is strictly prohibited. All rights reserved.
This content is provided for test preparation purposes only and does not imply an endorsement by Mometrix of any particular political, scientific, or religious point of view.

Patient Care

Ethical and Legal Aspects

Information to Collect from Patient Before Receiving Outpatient or Inpatient Services

The radiograph is not the only important part of a radiographic procedure. It is also important to obtain an accurate patient history when a radiographic procedure is conducted. It provides the radiologist with information necessary for accurately reading and interpreting the radiograph.

The information that should be collected from a patient before receiving services is as follows:

- Outpatient Services
  - Pregnancy information for women of childbearing age
  - Whether or not the patient did everything asked of them prior to the procedure
  - The reason that the patient is in for the procedure
  - Length of time that the patient has been experiencing problem
  - Visible signs of injury, illness, or pain/discomfort
  - Patient medications (particularly ones that may interfere with the image)
- Inpatient Services
  - Patient consent for the procedure
  - Date of any previous procedure
  - Labs and results relevant to the procedure
  - Medications that may adversely affect results (and prevent the procedure)
  - Patient condition that could prevent the procedure
  - Any patient information that may have an impact on the treatment

Patient Comfort

Radiographic procedures can be uncomfortable due to equipment and positioning. This can be made worse by the illness or injury of the patient. It is the responsibility of radiographic personnel to ease discomfort as much as possible. This includes the use of cushions, pillows, and sponges, as well as positioning considerations. A radiographer should also attend to basic patient needs such as allowing them going to the bathroom (and assisting when necessary), providing drinking water, warm blankets, a damp cloth, lip balm, and necessary personal cleanliness. If the patient is uncomfortable in any way, they are more likely to move and movement can compromise the quality of the image making a repeat procedure necessary. Thus, by making a patient as comfortable as possible, you enhance both the patient's experience and the quality of the image.

Informed Consent

Informed consent is communication between a patient and a healthcare provider that results in the patient giving the provider permission to perform a specific medical procedure. Informed consent means the patient has received comprehensive information about his or her diagnosis, the procedure to be performed, the risks of the procedure, alternatives to the procedure and their risks and the risks of not having the treatment or procedure. As part of informed consent, the patient should be permitted to ask questions to gain a thorough understanding of the recommended treatment. Informed consent is an ethical obligation and legal requirement in all 50 states.

Copyright © Mometrix Media. You have been licensed one copy of this document for personal use only. Any other reproduction or redistribution is strictly prohibited. All rights reserved.
This content is provided for test preparation purposes only and does not imply an endorsement by Mometrix of any particular political, scientific, or religious point of view.

Even if a physician writes a request to perform a radiological procedure, an informed consent is necessary before the procedure can be done. Legally, only a physician can get consent from the patient to do a procedure. This is because it is believed that it is the physician who is qualified to provide the patient with all of the necessary information (risks vs. benefits). This, however, is not always the case. It is still important for radiology personnel to provide the patient with thorough information regarding the procedure, particularly if there are any risks involved. With invasive or risky procedures, it is necessary to get written consent from the patient before the procedure is done.

Exceptions

There are some exceptions to the rule of informed consent. They are as follows:

- Emergencies: If the patient's life is at stake, they are unconscious, and the procedure is widely accepted a necessary for treatment, there is no need to get informed consent.
- Emotional Distress/not able to process information: Informed consent is not necessary if a patient is unable to understand the information given to him by the doctor, whether it is because of a mental handicap or the patient has become emotionally distraught.
- Legal Incompetence: Informed consent is waived if a judge rules a patient incompetent.
- Minor Age Status: Informed consent may be waived if the patient is a minor and getting parental consent is not a possibility. If the procedure is not a matter of life or death, it may be postponed until a legal guardian can consent to it.

Requirements

In order for a procedure to be performed, the ordering doctor must provide the patient with all necessary information and get their consent to have it done. The following are the requirements for getting informed consent for a procedure:

- The physician ordering the procedure got consent to do so from the patient.
- Risk/Benefit information was provided to the patient.
- Other treatment possibilities were discussed with patient.
- Patient informed of possible outcome if the procedure is not done.
- Patient was informed using understandable language.
- The place that provided the service also provided patient with information about risks.
- State-mandated rules regarding time between signing consent and performing procedure were followed.
- The patient was not scared or forced into having the procedure performed.

Confidentiality and Diagnosis/Interpretation

The American Society of Radiological Technologists has developed a code of ethics that acts as a guideline for the radiographer in completing their job in the best possible manner. Confidentiality and diagnosis/interpretation are important aspects of this code of ethics. It is the responsibility of the radiographer to respect a patient's privacy and confidentiality. This includes any information about the procedure, diagnosis, medical or personal history. The only exception to this policy is legally required information. It is also the responsibility of the radiographer to understand the scope and limitations of their profession. It is absolutely not the job of a radiographer to provide interpretations or diagnosis. Even if years of experience yield extensive knowledge and abilities, the radiographer should never overstep these bounds.

Copyright © Mometrix Media. You have been licensed one copy of this document for personal use only. Any other reproduction or redistribution is strictly prohibited. All rights reserved.
This content is provided for test preparation purposes only and does not imply an endorsement by Mometrix of any particular political, scientific, or religious point of view.

HIPAA

HIPAA is the Health Insurance Portability and Accountability Act approved by congress and signed into law in 1996. HIPAA was enacted to protect the privacy of personal health information by setting limits on the use and disclosure of such information without patient authorization. The Act also gives patients' rights over their health information, including the right to examine and obtain copies of their health records and the right to request corrections.

Patient Privacy

Every patient has a right to privacy during a procedure. The basics of patient privacy for a radiographic procedure are as follows:

- Provide a private area for changing or dressing.
- Provide a dressing gown that has closures (use two gowns if the patient is large).
- Cover the patients' exposed legs and feet. Provide slippers if necessary.
- Only expose parts of the body that are necessary for the procedure.
- Allow only necessary personnel in the room during the procedure.
- Do not have personal conversations with other personnel in front of the patient.
- Show the patient's chart to only necessary personnel and do not discuss the patient with others.
- Respect patient confidentiality.

Patient's Rights

Even if a physician writes an order to perform a procedure, it is ultimately up to the patient to decide if the procedure will be performed. Every patient has the right to refuse any medical procedure. This patient's right, among others, stems from the Patient's Bill of Rights. In 1973, the American Hospital Association developed the first Patient's Bill of Rights. It was a document that outlined a patient's rights when it comes to choices in healthcare. This Bill of rights has been updated and adopted, in some form, by most states, and it is the responsibility of the radiographer to become familiar with their local version. It covers topics such as informed consent, advanced directives, living wills, appointment of surrogates, confidentiality, privacy, access to medical records, and access to healthcare.

Advance Directives

In accordance to Federal and state laws, individuals have the right to self-determination in health care, including decisions about end of life care through **advance directives** such as living wills and the right to assign a surrogate person to make decisions through a durable power of attorney. Patients should routinely be questioned about an advanced directive as they may present at a healthcare provider without the document. Patients who have indicated they desire a do-not-resuscitate (DNR) order should not receive resuscitative treatments for terminal illness or conditions in which meaningful recovery cannot occur. Patients and families of those with terminal illnesses should be questioned as to whether the patients are Hospice patients. For those with DNR requests or those withdrawing life support, staff should provide the patient palliative rather than curative measures, such as pain control and/or oxygen, and emotional support to the patient and family. Religious traditions and beliefs about death should be treated with respect.

Beneficence and Nonmaleficence

Beneficence is an ethical principle that involves performing actions that are for the purpose of benefitting another person. In the care of a patient, any procedure or treatment should be done with the ultimate goal of benefitting the patient, and any actions that are not beneficial should be

Copyright © Mometrix Media. You have been licensed one copy of this document for personal use only. Any other reproduction or redistribution is strictly prohibited. All rights reserved.
This content is provided for test preparation purposes only and does not imply an endorsement by Mometrix of any particular political, scientific, or religious point of view.

reconsidered. As conditions change, procedures need to be continually reevaluated to determine if they are still of benefit.

Nonmaleficence is an ethical principle that means healthcare workers should provide care in a manner that does not cause direct intentional harm to the patient:

- The actual act must be good or morally neutral.
- The intent must be only for a good effect.
- A bad effect cannot serve as the means to get to a good effect.
- A good effect must have more benefit than a bad effect has harm.

Requirements for Research Participation

Research participation requires precise documentation for every step, not only for the subject's safety and rights but also to protect the validity of the study being conducted. The pretrial documentation should include the brochures for the trial and how they recruited subjects, compensation, certificates that outline how products will be shipped along with their purity, and signed consent forms. During the trial, standard operation procedure (SOP) and specific protocols should be in place along with the confidential list of participants and any records pertaining to the patient's care (e.g., prescriptions, labs, radiology exams, and notes kept by the subject). After the trial, a case study is produced explaining the results of the trial. It is communicated if subjects will need follow-up care, and all supplies are accounted for and returned to the vendor. All of the documentation should be the original paperwork that was filed during the trial. If the original files cannot be provided, a certified copy should be used. The paperwork should also have signatures to identify who filed the paperwork along with the dates.

Risk Management in Relation to Legal and Professional Responsibilities

Because of all of the potential legal issues regarding negligence within the medical field, risk management has become an important way for medical institutions to minimize liability and risk. Incident reports are used to document any problems or questionable incidents that occur in a department. If an incident report is filed, it does not necessarily mean that a person is admitting guilt or that supervisors view the staff involved as guilty. It is simply a clear and consistent way to document just what happened in an incident that has the potential for future investigation. If anything, it can protect medical personnel if a patient charges negligence.

TQI and TQM in Relation to Legal and Professional Responsibilities

TQI (total quality improvement) and TQM (total quality management) are ways to measure and manage the quality of service as a means to reduce liability and risk. They look at the quality of service as a function of productivity. Many businesses, not just healthcare, use TQI and TQM to improve quality and productivity. In healthcare, it is a way to cut costs without sacrificing service. It does not, however, take into consideration the human nature of healthcare. Every patient is different and has different needs. It is important that the radiographer follows department protocol for quality improvement and productivity, but always keeps in mind individual patient needs and the code of ethics.

Request to Perform an Examination

Before any radiographic procedure is conducted, it is necessary to have a formal request from a doctor. The request may be written, faxed, or verbal. The submission of a request is the first step in a radiological procedure. The request should include all of the necessary patient information such as name, age, date of birth, medical number, patient type, date of last menstrual period (when appropriate), the physician, and the type of procedure to be done. This last bit of information is,

Copyright © Mometrix Media. You have been licensed one copy of this document for personal use only. Any other reproduction or redistribution is strictly prohibited. All rights reserved.
This content is provided for test preparation purposes only and does not imply an endorsement by Mometrix of any particular political, scientific, or religious point of view.

perhaps, the most important. Without it, the radiographer does not know what needs to be done. If there is any question regarding the order, it is the responsibility of the radiographer to contact the ordering physician to get a clarification.

Proper Patient Identification

Proper patient identification is important because it can prevent a critical error like misidentifying a patient specimen which could result in harm or death to a patient. Patient identification includes asking a patient to state their name and date of birth, and then you check the identification band and the requisition to see if they match. Verbal identification should never be relied on alone although it is important since patients can be hard of hearing, ill, or mentally incompetent and may give incorrect information. Also, check the identification band since it is possible for a patient to be wearing the wrong ID band. If there is no ID band, notify the nurse and have her confirm the patient's identity and attach an ID band before the blood is drawn. If there is any discrepancy on the ID band, information given by the patient or on the requisition, a reconciliation of the discrepancy must be made before a collection is taken. More than one patient may have the same name. Usually a name alert is placed on the chart but not in all cases.

Negligence

There are four parts to negligent behavior: duty, breach of duty, causation, damages. Behavior is termed negligent when a radiographer does not correctly or adequately perform a previously outlined duty that results in harm (or potential harm) to the patient. The key is that the duty must be defined. If harm befalls a patient while under the care of a radiographer, their actions will be carefully analyzed to see if there was any negligence on the part of the radiographer. Even if no harm befalls a patient, a radiographer can be considered negligent if proper procedure has not been followed and there was a potential for harm. Thus, it is not only important that the radiographer is well informed of proper procedure, but that the procedure is followed.

Civil Liability

It is the ethical and legal responsibility of the radiographer to do their job in an accurate and professional manner. If not, the radiographer may be held responsible for negligence and be demanded by the courts to compensate the patient for damages. This responsibility is referred to as civil liability and is determined by a series of intentional torts (civil wrongs done on purpose with the intent to interfere with a person's physical freedom). Intentional torts are battery (not getting consent from the patient to touch them, acting in a way that injures or harms the patient), assault (threatening an uncooperative patient), false imprisonment (unnecessarily restraining a patient), intentional infliction of emotional distress (extreme behavior that causes emotional distress), and defamation (providing false information about a patient).

Subpoena Duces Tecum

Subpoena duces tecum literally means bring [it] with you under penalty of punishment. It is a court order for a witness to produce documents. The judge must carefully consider if *subpoena duces tecum* transgresses the patient's HIPAA rights.

Handling Wounds of Violence and Child Abuse

The physician and other health professionals must report to authorities:

- Gunshot wounds
- Possible terrorist incidents, especially if they involve the spread of disease
- Known or suspected abuse of a child, senior, or disabled person
- Sexual assault of a juvenile or disabled person

Copyright © Mometrix Media. You have been licensed one copy of this document for personal use only. Any other reproduction or redistribution is strictly prohibited. All rights reserved.
This content is provided for test preparation purposes only and does not imply an endorsement by Mometrix of any particular political, scientific, or religious point of view.

- Poisoning
- Wounds intentionally caused by knives and sharp objects
- Criminal violence, including domestic violence
- Client-specific information for the central cancer registry
- Specific contagious diseases determined by each state

Good Samaritan Act and Duty of Care

There are two kinds of Good Samaritan Acts:

- A first aider who provides unpaid assistance to the injured in an emergency and acts as "a reasonable man" up to his/her level of training is protected by state law from unfair prosecution for death, disability, or disfigurement. A judge would dismiss assault and battery charges. A *Good Samaritan Act* is not a duty to assist law, except in Vermont and Minnesota. Nevada and California may adopt a duty to assist clause.
- A living donor who offers a non-directed donation of an organ to the transplant center is a Good Samaritan. The following organs can be donated by a living donor: kidneys; liver lobes; lung lobes; pancreas segments; and small bowel segments. Non-direct donors do not have anyone particular in mind whom they would like to receive their donated organ. The donation is usually anonymous and the Good Samaritan is blameless for complications the recipient suffers.

Duty of care: One must act as "a reasonable man" and meet the standard of care to avoid negligence charges. This means being watchful, attentive, cautious, and prudent at work.

Restraints

Restraint policies vary from one facility to another, but their purpose remains the same.

- Restraints are applied in order to protect the patient from causing harm to himself or to other people.
- A restraint may be applied to prevent the patient from interfering with medical devices or moving in a way that would be detrimental to his health.
- It may also be applied if the patient is showing signs of aggression.
- A restraint should always be applied after all other alternatives have been exhausted.

It should not be applied as a form of punishment or for the convenience of the staff.

Prior to applying a restraint, all other alternatives must be exhausted. The health care staff must attempt to identify and address the behaviors that require the application of restraints.

- An order from the patient's physician must be obtained in order to apply restraints, and the physician should visibly assess the patient within 24 hours of the time of application of the restraints.
- Consent should be obtained from the patient's next of kin.
- Care must be taken to choose the least restrictive form of restraint.
- The type of restraint should be explained to the patient, as well as the reasons for the application of the restraint and the requirements for removal of the restraint.

Copyright © Mometrix Media. You have been licensed one copy of this document for personal use only. Any other reproduction or redistribution is strictly prohibited. All rights reserved.
This content is provided for test preparation purposes only and does not imply an endorsement by Mometrix of any particular political, scientific, or religious point of view.

Alternatives

There are a number of measures that can be performed as an alternative to applying restraints. The type of alternatives that are utilized may vary depending upon the patient. Any needs should be assessed and all reasonable alternatives performed prior to application of restraints.

- The patient may need to be moved to a quiet environment.
- He may require more stimulation, such as hearing a television or radio in the background.
- He may require redirection.
- The patient may need toileting or water.
- He may need personal items placed within reach.
- He may require distraction if the care team is attempting to remove a medical device.
- If the patient has an illness or requires rest, it may cause him to act in a manner that is confused or inappropriate.

Applying Restraints to Extremities

Extremity restraints are applied to the arms and legs to restrict movement. A doctor's order and consent from the family must be obtained prior to application of these restraints.

- The nurse aide should wash her hands and don a pair of gloves.
- She should greet the patient and explain the need for the restraint, as well as the requirements for removal.
- The restraint should be applied per the manufacturer's instructions and tied to the frame of the bed using a quick release knot.
- The patient should be given a reasonable amount of slack in order to move.
- The nurse aide should be able to fit two fingers between the patient's extremity and the restraint; this ensures that is it not too tight.

Monitoring Patients

Patients who are in restraints should be closely monitored to ensure safety.

- They should be checked every 30 minutes to make sure there is proper circulation.
- While they are restrained, patients should have their legs covered with a blanket in order to maintain privacy.
- The restraint should be removed every 2 hours to allow for range of motion.
- Patients should also be repositioned for comfort and offered water and toileting every two hours.
- Teaching regarding the restraints should be frequently reinforced to encourage patient understanding of the need for the restraint and the requirements for removal.

Securing Restraints to a Wheelchair Versus a Bed

When securing restraints on a patient who is in a wheelchair, care should be taken to ensure the restraint is tied using a quick release knot attached directly to the frame of the wheelchair. The wheelchair should be locked, and care should be taken to ensure the restraints are not tied to the wheels.

Similarly, when the patient is in bed, the restraint should be tied using a quick release knot attached directly to the frame of the bed. Tying the restraint to the side rail can cause injury to the patient if the side rail should fall.

Copyright © Mometrix Media. You have been licensed one copy of this document for personal use only. Any other reproduction or redistribution is strictly prohibited. All rights reserved.
This content is provided for test preparation purposes only and does not imply an endorsement by Mometrix of any particular political, scientific, or religious point of view.

Types

There are a number of different types of restraints that can be used in a health care setting.

- Emotional restraints are a method of using verbal or emotional cues in order to attempt to modify the patient's behaviors. This can include limit setting or contracting with the patient for safety.
- Environmental restraints are devices used to restrict patient movement. These include side-rails on the bed or locked doors within the facility. When all four side-rails are in a raised position on the bed, it is considered to be a restraint.
- Physical restraints are devices that can be applied to the patient to restrict movement. These include wrist and vest restraints, lap belts, and movement pads.
- Chemical restraints are medications that are given to the patient to modify behavior.

Vest Restraints

A vest restraint is a device that is placed over the patient's chest to restrict movement. It is typically applied to prevent a patient from getting up without assistance. A doctor's order and consent from the family must be obtained prior to application of the restraint.

- The nurse aide should wash her hands and don a pair of gloves.
- She should greet the patient and explain the need for the restraint, as well as the requirements for removal.
- The vest restraint should be placed on the patient so that the opening is toward the back, with the straps crossing in the back.
- The straps should then be tied with a quick release knot directly to the chair or the frame of the bed.
- At least two fingers should be able to fit beneath the vest restraint to ensure that it is not too tight.
- Once the restraint has been applied, remove the gloves and wash your hands.
- Monitor the patient per facility policy.

Immobilization of Patient During CT

The positioning and immobilization of the patient during CT is crucial if the practitioner is to obtain an accurate reading. The positioning should be conducive to replication because the treatment machine can reproduce the virtual simulation parameters in the event that a follow-up or second screening becomes necessary. Devices provided for immobilization and registered to the treatment table allow practitioners to position the patient correctly for the different scans required for each study, usually ranging from 100 to 200 scans. Diagnostic CT scanners are fitted with external laser alignment systems and virtual simulation software that allow practitioners to study the patient from a beam's eye view (BEV) and a room's eye view (REV) display. Digitally reconstructed radiographs (DRRs), multiplanar reformatted images (MPRs), and digitally composited radiographs (DCRs) can also be produced by the CT scanner, although these technological advances are not useful if the patient is not properly immobilized during the test.

Potential Legal Issues Regarding Manipulation of Electronic Data

Exams performed in the radiology department are part of the patient's legal file (whether they are captured on film or digital equipment). To provide the correct diagnosis for a patient the technologist must make sure that the name of the patient is on the film as well as the date. Technologists must verify they have the correct patient prior to performing any exam. Another legal requirement is that technologists must utilize their lead markers with their identifying initials

Copyright © Mometrix Media. You have been licensed one copy of this document for personal use only. Any other reproduction or redistribution is strictly prohibited. All rights reserved.
This content is provided for test preparation purposes only and does not imply an endorsement by Mometrix of any particular political, scientific, or religious point of view.

on the films even if using equipment. It is important to use collimation as any digital masking or shuttering performed after the exposure has been taken may not be admissible in court. It is important that the technologist doesn't rely on post-processing techniques to create an image. Technologists must be even more cautious of the as low as reasonably achievable (ALARA) principle when using digital radiography equipment. Extensive knowledge of techniques is important so that one does not overexpose patients. Technologists should be familiar with acceptable exposure indicator ranges for the different vendors used in a department.

Principles of ASRT Code of Ethics

The American Society of Radiological Technologists has developed a code of ethics that acts as a guideline for the radiographer in completing their job in the best possible manner. The ten principles of this code of ethics are as follows:

- Act in a professional manner.
- Respect the dignity of everyone.
- Deliver healthcare without discrimination.
- Be a competent technician.
- Make decisions that take into consideration the needs of your patients.
- Diagnosis and interpretation are not your job or responsibility.
- Be aware of and practice current technical and safety procedures.
- Practice ethical behavior that provides quality care.
- Respect patient privacy and confidentiality.
- Be involved in continuing education.

Important Terms

DNR: Do not resuscitate. No codes should be called for this patient and no heroic measures should be taken to revive patient if the patient stops breathing.

NPO: From the Latin phrase nil per os meaning nothing by mouth. Patients are not allowed food or drink including water. This restriction is usually placed on a patient before and after a procedure.

STAT: From the Latin word statim means immediately. It describes the need for a specimen or test to be done immediately in response to critical situations with the possibility of the test results preventing a patient's death.

ASAP: As soon as possible, this is used if the results are needed soon but not to prevent the patient from dying

Fasting: When a person refrains from eating or drinking anything before a procedure, sometimes water is allowed on a fast

Statute of Limitations: A law defining the maximum period the complainant or appellant can wait before filing a lawsuit. The limitation date varies according to the type of case and if it falls within state or federal jurisdiction. Usually, the limitation is 1 to 6 years. Homicide has no limitation. If the complainant misses the deadline, then the right to sue is "stats barred" (dead). Rarely, a judge will "toll" (extend) the deadline if the injury was discovered late or a trusted person hid misuse of funds or failure to pay. Minors' rights to bring negligence charges are tolled until the age of 18.

Assumption of Risk: (A.) A defense against an accusation of negligence. The defendant states the situation was obviously hazardous, so the complainant should have realized injury could result. (B.)

Copyright © Mometrix Media. You have been licensed one copy of this document for personal use only. Any other reproduction or redistribution is strictly prohibited. All rights reserved.
This content is provided for test preparation purposes only and does not imply an endorsement by Mometrix of any particular political, scientific, or religious point of view.

An insurance company takes the risk of extending coverage, realizing the policyholder might make a claim, but it is statistically more likely to make a profit from the premiums.

Arbitration Agreement: The patient agrees to give up the right to sue the doctor. An arbiter (arbitrator) awards damages if injury results. Settlement is faster for the patient, and the doctor gets a malpractice insurance discount. Both parties save on legal fees.

Negligence: Taking an unreasonable, careless action that could foreseeably cause harm. Failing to exercise due care for others that a prudent, reasonable person would do. Negligence is accidental. Negligence is not an intentional tort, such as trespass or assault. Business errors, miscalculations, and failure to act can be negligent.

Contributory Negligence: If a person is injured partially because of his/her own negligence: even if it is slight: then the person who caused the accident does not pay any damages (money) to the injured person. Forty-four states recognize that applying the rule of contributory negligence could lead to unfair acquittal of genuinely negligent defendants, so they now use a comparative negligence test as a more balanced approach. In the 6 states that still have contributory negligence rules, juries tend to ignore it as unfair.

Comparative Negligence: A rule used in accident cases to calculate the percentage of responsibility of each person (joint tortfeasors) directly involved in the accident. Damages (money compensation) are awarded based on a complex formula.

Defamation: Defaming a person exposes him or her to public ridicule or tarnishes his or her memory through untrue and malicious statements. The defamed person can lose business due to loss of his or her good name.

Slander: Oral statements that damage someone's reputation. It is a form of defamation.

Libel: A written statement that harms an individual's character, name, or reputation. A defamatory libel statement may be true, but is published maliciously (without just cause).

Invasion of Privacy: Unsolicited or unauthorized exposure of patient information.

Malpractice: Professional misconduct, resulting in failure to provide due care. Most malpractice lawsuits are related to professional negligence, the failure to perform what is considered standard care.

Fraud: Intentional dishonesty for unfair or illegal gain.

Assault and Battery: Assault is declaring or threatening your intent to touch a patient inappropriately or to cause physical harm. Battery is the actual act of inappropriate touching.

Subpoena: A legal writ (order) requiring a person to come to court, to testify in court, and/or to produce documents or evidence. Failure to do so may result in fine or jailing.

Res Ipsa Loquitur ("the thing speaks for itself"): The principle of law that allows the use of circumstantial evidence as proof.

Locum tenens ("to substitute for"): Allows one medical professional to serve temporarily in place of another. For example, a physician's practice may be covered by another physician usually for a few days up to 6 months when the first goes on vacation or takes leave. Companies specialize in providing locums physicians to work on a contract basis.

Copyright © Mometrix Media. You have been licensed one copy of this document for personal use only. Any other reproduction or redistribution is strictly prohibited. All rights reserved.
This content is provided for test preparation purposes only and does not imply an endorsement by Mometrix of any particular political, scientific, or religious point of view.

Deposition: This is a sworn out-of-court witness statement taken under oath, usually in an attorney's office prior to a court case to document what the witness knows and to preserve the statements for use in court.

Stare Decisis ("to stand on the decisions"): It expresses the common law doctrine that court decisions should be guided by precedent.

Respondeat Superior ("let the master answer"): A doctrine in tort law that makes a master liable for the wrong of a servant; specifically, the doctrine making an employer or principal liable for the wrong of an employee or agent if it was committed within the scope of employment or agency.

Communicable Infection: An illness caused by the direct or indirect transmission of a specific infectious agent or the toxins it produces from an infected person, animal, or inanimate host to a susceptible body; indirect transmission can be via a vector, intermediate plant or animal host, or the inanimate environment.

Nosocomial Infection: Hospital-acquired illness not resulting from the original reason for the patient to be admitted.

Lumen: Lumen is the hollow area within a blood vessel

Valves: Valves are tissue flaps inside a vein or the heart that prevent backward flow of blood. Valves open as blood moves through them and close under the weight of blood collecting in the vein due to decreased pressure and gravity.

Interpersonal Communication

Verbal and Nonverbal Modes of Communicating

Because the radiographer is usually the only person to have contact with a patient during a radiographic procedure, it is important that they effectively communicate all important information, collect the necessary patient history, as well as make the patient feel as comfortable as possible. This is all done using various verbal and nonverbal modes of communication. The verbal ways that we communicate with others are obvious-we ask questions, provide information, clarify misunderstandings. Some of the ways that we communicate nonverbally are less obvious, yet equally as important. Nonverbal communication ranges from the organization and cleanliness of the radiographer and the radiography room, to the ways in which the patient is touched or transferred for the procedure. It is important to convey to the patient an attitude of understanding, caring, and competency.

Importance of Nonverbal Communication

Any type of message transmitted between two people that does not involve words is nonverbal communication. 85% to 93% of successful communication depends on nonverbal cues. Remember that your patient is likely apprehensive and English may not be his/her first language. Your patient may have difficulty speaking due to injury, drugs, age, deformity, developmental disability, or the instruments used during a procedure. Watch your patient's facial expressions, gestures, posture, and position. Tight posture and/or crossed arms and legs suggest resistance. Conversely, relaxed posture and uncrossed appendages suggest openness. Your posture affects your patient. Sit closely beside your patient, rather than towering directly over him/her in an intimidating manner. Explain what you are going to do. A patient feels more comfortable when he/she is well informed. Maintain the proper social distance (territoriality) between yourself and your patient during discussions (about 3 feet apart).

Copyright © Mometrix Media. You have been licensed one copy of this document for personal use only. Any other reproduction or redistribution is strictly prohibited. All rights reserved.
This content is provided for test preparation purposes only and does not imply an endorsement by Mometrix of any particular political, scientific, or religious point of view.

Cultural Considerations with Patients

Hispanic Patients

Many areas of the country have large populations of **Hispanic** and Hispanic-Americans. As always, it's important to recognize that cultural generalizations don't always apply to individuals. Recent immigrants, especially, have cultural needs that the nurse must understand:

- Many Hispanics are Catholic and may like the nurse to make arrangements for a priest to visit.
- Large extended families may come to visit to support the patient and family, so patients should receive clear explanations about how many visitors are allowed, but some flexibility may be required.
- Language barriers may exist as some may have limited or no English skills so translation services should be available around the clock.
- Hispanic culture encourages outward expressions of emotions, so family may react strongly to news about a patient's condition, and people who are ill may expect some degree of pampering, so extra attention to the patient/family members may alleviate some of their anxiety.

Cultural Considerations with Hispanic Patients

Caring for **Hispanic** and Hispanic-American patients requires understanding of cultural differences:

- Some immigrant Hispanics have very little formal education, so medical information may seem very complex and confusing, and they may not understand the implications or need for follow-up care.
- Hispanic culture perceives time with more flexibility than American, so if parents need to be present at a particular time, the nurse should specify the exact time (1:30 PM) and explain the reason rather than saying something more vague, such as "after lunch."
- People may appear to be unassertive or unable to make decisions when they are simply showing respect to the nurse by being deferent.
- In traditional families, the males make decisions, so a woman waits for the father or other males in the family to make decisions about treatment or care.
- Families may choose to use folk medicines instead of Western medical care or may combine the two.
- Children and young women are often sheltered and are taught to be respectful to adults, so they may not express their needs openly.

Middle Eastern Patients

Caring for **Middle Eastern** patients requires understanding of cultural differences:

- Families may practice strict dietary restrictions, such as avoiding pork and requiring that animals be killed in a ritual manner, so vegetarian or kosher meals may be required.
- People may have language difficulties requiring a translator, and same-sex translators should be used if at all possible.
- Families may be accompanied by large extended families that want to be kept informed and whom patients consult before decisions are made.
- Most medical care is provided by female relatives, so educating the family about patient care should be directed at females (with female translators if necessary).
- Outward expressions of grief are considered as showing respect for the dead.

Copyright © Mometrix Media. You have been licensed one copy of this document for personal use only. Any other reproduction or redistribution is strictly prohibited. All rights reserved.
This content is provided for test preparation purposes only and does not imply an endorsement by Mometrix of any particular political, scientific, or religious point of view.

- Middle Eastern families often offer gifts to caregivers. Small gifts (candy) that can be shared should be accepted graciously, but for other gifts, the families should be advised graciously that accepting gifts is against hospital policy.
- Middle Easterners often require less personal space and may stand very close.

Cultural Considerations with Middle Eastern Patients

There are considerable cultural differences among **Middle Easterners,** but religious beliefs about the segregation of males and females are common. It's important to remember that segregating the female is meant to protect her virtue. Female nurses have low status in many countries because they violate this segregation by touching male bodies, so parents may not trust or show respect for the nurse who is caring for their family member. Additionally, male patients may not want to be cared for by female nurses or doctors, and families may be very upset at a female being cared for by a male nurse or physician. When possible, these cultural traditions should be accommodated:

- In Middle Eastern countries, males make decisions, so issues for discussion or decision should be directed to males, such as the father or spouse, and males may be direct in stating what they want, sometimes appearing demanding.
- If a male nurse must care for a female patient, then the family should be advised that *personal care* (such as bathing) will be done by a female while the medical treatments will be done by the male nurse.

Asian Patients

Caring for **Asian** patients requires understanding of cultural differences:

- Patients/families may not show outward expressions of feelings/grief, sometimes appearing passive. They also avoid public displays of affection. This does not mean that they don't feel, just that they don't show their feelings.
- Families often hide illness and disabilities from others and may feel ashamed about illness.
- Terminal illness is often hidden from the patient, so families may not want patients to know they are dying or seriously ill.
- Families may use cupping, pinching, or applying pressure to injured areas, and this can leave bruises that may appear as abuse, so when bruises are found, the family should be questioned about alternative therapy before assumptions are made.
- Patients may be treated with traditional herbs.
- Families may need translators because of poor or no English skills.
- In traditional Asian families, males are authoritative and make the decisions.

Cultural Considerations with Asian Patients

There are considerable differences among different **Asian** populations, so cultural generalizations may not apply to all, but nurses caring for Asian patients should be aware of common cultural attitudes and behaviors:

- Nurses and doctors are viewed with respect, so traditional Asian families may expect the nurse to remain authoritative and to give directions and may not question, so the nurse should ensure that they understand by having them review material or give demonstrations and should provide explanations clearly, anticipating questions that the family might have but may not articulate.

Copyright © Mometrix Media. You have been licensed one copy of this document for personal use only. Any other reproduction or redistribution is strictly prohibited. All rights reserved.
This content is provided for test preparation purposes only and does not imply an endorsement by Mometrix of any particular political, scientific, or religious point of view.

- Disagreeing is considered impolite. "Yes" may only mean that the person is heard, not that they agree with the person. When asked if they understand, they may indicate that they do even when they clearly do not so as not to offend the nurse.
- Asians may avoid eye contact as an indication of respect. This is especially true of children in relation to adults and younger adults in relation to elders.

Cultural Competence

Different cultures view health and illness from very different perspectives, and patients often come from a mix of many cultures, so the acute care nurse must be not only accepting of cultural differences but must be sensitive and aware. There are a number of characteristics that are important for a nurse to have **cultural competence:**

- **Appreciating diversity:** This must be grounded in information about other cultures and understanding of their value system.
- **Assessing own cultural perspectives:** Self-awareness is essential to understanding potential biases.
- **Understanding intercultural dynamics:** This must include understanding ways in which cultures cooperate, differ, communicate, and reach understanding.
- **Recognizing institutional culture:** Each institutional unit (hospital, clinic, office) has an inherent set of values that may be unwritten but is accepted by the staff.
- **Adapting patient service to diversity:** This is the culmination of cultural competence as it is the point of contact between cultures.

Administration of Blood Products and Jehovah Witnesses

Jehovah Witnesses have traditionally shunned transfusions and blood products as part of their religious belief. In 2004, the *Watchtower,* a Jehovah Witness publication presented a guide for members. When medical care indicates the need for blood transfusion or blood products and the patient and/or family members are practicing Jehovah Witnesses, this may present a conflict. It's important to approach the patient/family with full information and reasons for the transfusion or blood components without being judgmental, allowing them to express their feelings. In fact, studies show that while adults often refuse transfusions for themselves, they frequently allow their children to receive blood products, so one should never assume that an individual would refuse blood products based on the religion alone. Jehovah Witnesses can receive fractionated blood cells, thus allowing hemoglobin-based blood substitutes.

Basic blood standards for Jehovah Witnesses:

- ***Not acceptable:*** Whole blood: red cells, white cells, platelets, plasma
- ***Acceptable:*** Fractions from red cells, white cells, platelets, and plasma

Therapeutic Communication Techniques

Hearing Impaired Patients

Hearing impaired patients may have some hearing and may use hearing aids while **deaf** patients typically have little or no hearing. Some patients are able to use lip reading to various degrees, so one should always face the patient (at 3-6 feet) and speak slowly and clearly, using gestures (not excessively) to augment speech:

- Hearing impaired: Assistive devices (hearing aids, writing material) should be available and used during communication. Use a normal tone of voice and speak in short sentences. Minimize environmental noises.

Copyright © Mometrix Media. You have been licensed one copy of this document for personal use only. Any other reproduction or redistribution is strictly prohibited. All rights reserved.
This content is provided for test preparation purposes only and does not imply an endorsement by Mometrix of any particular political, scientific, or religious point of view.

- Deaf: If patients are deaf, sign language interpreters should be used for important communication (face the patient, not the interpreter). Assistive devices, such as writing materials, TDD phone/relay service, should be available for use. Always announce presence on entering a room by waving, clapping, tapping the foot (whatever works best for the patient). Ensure alarms have visual feedback (lights). Do not chew, smoke, or eat while speaking to the patient.

Visually Impaired Patients

Visual impairment is unrelated to intelligence or hearing, so one should speak with age-appropriate vocabulary in a normal tone of voice, facing the patient so one can observe facial expression. Depending on the degree of visual impairment the patient may not be able to see gestures or materials, so alternate forms of materials (braille handouts or enlarged text) or manipulatives must be considered. The field of vision may be impaired so that the patient sees shapes or has better vision in some areas than others, and one should try to position herself/himself for the patient's advantage. One should also announce his/her presence, explain actions and movement ("I'm putting your dressing supplies on the counter."), announce position ("I'm at your right side.") and always tell the patient if intending to touch the patient ("I'm going to take your blood pressure on your right arm").

Effective Communication with the Intellectually Disabled and Illiterate

Communicating with patients who are **intellectually disabled** can be challenging, and patients may have very different and individual responses, so observation of the patient must serve as a guide. Patients may be apprehensive and frightened, so one should maintain a friendly normal tone of voice and should speak with the patient often to establish rapport, even if the response is not clear. One should always ask the patient before touching his/her things. Initiating communication by talking about familiar things (family, pictures, the past) may be comforting for the patient. If responses are unclear or inappropriate, one can say, "I didn't understand that" but should not laugh or indicate frustration. Communicating with patients who are **illiterate** is not different than with most patients because the patients may be quite intelligent, but one should take care to explain procedures and provide verbal rather than written instructions.

Therapeutic Responses to Various Populations

Therapeutic responses include:

- Pediatric/Adolescent: Use vocabulary appropriate to age and encourage adolescents to make decisions whenever possible ("Which arm should I use?"). Avoid approaching young children too abruptly but chat with the child and caregiver to ease the child's fear. Explain in advance any actions to be taken, such as temperature or BP, and allow the child to see and hold the equipment when possible.
- Geriatric: Treat patients with respect, address them by their names ("Mrs. Jones") and avoid terms like "honey," and "dear." Be alert for barriers, such as hearing deficit, to communication, and encourage patients to ask questions and discuss concerns. Avoid rushing and interrupting and utilize active listening skills.
- Terminally ill: Avoid being excessively sympathetic ("You poor thing"), but remain patient and empathetic. Utilize active listening and allow patient time to express feelings or concerns. Understand that patients may be in pain, weak, frightened, nauseated, and/or depressed and may over-react or under-react.

Copyright © Mometrix Media. You have been licensed one copy of this document for personal use only. Any other reproduction or redistribution is strictly prohibited. All rights reserved.
This content is provided for test preparation purposes only and does not imply an endorsement by Mometrix of any particular political, scientific, or religious point of view.

Explaining Procedures to Patients

It is very important that the patient fully understands the procedure that is to be done. A patient cannot be expected to consent to a procedure that they do not understand. There are different ways that a radiographer can communicate the information to the patient. Because everyone has a different level of education and understanding of medical procedures, a radiographer must tailor their explanation to the patient's needs. The following steps should be taken to assure that the patient is adequately informed:

- Ask is the patient is familiar with the procedure.
- Find out if the procedure has already been explained to them.
- Provide a simple and concise explanation using language they will understand.
- Explain if the patient is to do anything during the procedure (not move, hold breath).
- Have the patient explain any important instructions back to you.
- Allow the patient to ask questions.

Communication Techniques When Assessing Understanding

Communication techniques used when assessing patient's understanding and communication include:

- Reflection: Refers to both the meaning of the patient's words and the emotions. If a patient states, "I understand how to monitor my blood pressure," a reflecting question might be: "You feel confident that you know how to take your blood pressure and when to notify the physician?"
- Restatement: Restates or paraphrases something a patient said, "I've been having dizzy spells for two weeks?" Restatement might be: "You've been having dizzy spells for 2 weeks."
- Clarification: Asks for more information. If a patient states, "I haven't been feeling well," a clarifying question might be: "What exactly do you mean when you say you haven't been feeling well?"
- Feedback: Responds to something a patient has said or done, letting them know that the message/information was received: "You have kept very accurate records of your blood pressure and pulse."

Common Internal and External Distractions That Disrupt Communication

Distractions (interference) that disrupt the communication cycle include:

- Internal: The communicator's or recipient's emotional status, such as increased anxiety or anger, can negatively impact communication. Biases, prejudices, and belief systems may also interfere with a person's ability to attend to the ideas of another person. Pain and hunger can be so distracting that the person is unable to focus on communication. When under stress, the brain may process information differently, interfering with comprehension.
- External: Noise in the environment (conversation, traffic, alarms, air conditioning) can make it hard for some people to hear clearly, especially those with hearing impairment, and may make concentration difficult. Additionally, people may find noise very stressful to the point that they have difficulty thinking. Other environmental factors, such as extremes of heat or cold, may cause physical discomfort that interferes with the ability to communicate.

Copyright © Mometrix Media. You have been licensed one copy of this document for personal use only. Any other reproduction or redistribution is strictly prohibited. All rights reserved.
This content is provided for test preparation purposes only and does not imply an endorsement by Mometrix of any particular political, scientific, or religious point of view.

Communication Techniques to Encourage in Therapeutic Relationships

The following are 4 *appropriate* communication techniques to encourage in therapeutic relationships:

- **Use active listening** – Paraphrase and repeat back information transmitted by your patient. Ask for clarification when the message is confusing. Summarize what you agreed to at the end of your conversation.
- **Watch for nonverbal cues** – Nonverbal cues are gestures, grimaces, posturing, appearance, and eye movements that comprise 85% of all communication. Nonverbal cues denote pain, fear, lying, depression, or subterfuge by a caregiver. Gently ask your patient to clarify when verbal and nonverbal cues do not match. Children and psychiatric patients may develop tic disorders (involuntary gestures and movements). If you cannot decipher which movements are truly cues and which are tics, ask the doctor.
- **Ask open-ended questions** – Get your patient to 'open up', rather than ask questions that require only a yes or no answer.
- **Consider influences** – Put communication in the context of your patient's: Developmental age; emotions; values; ethics; health; education; culture; environment; social and family status; and drug levels.

Inappropriate Communications Techniques

The following are 10 *inappropriate* communications techniques to avoid in therapeutic relationships:

- **Ask leading questions** – Never shape the patient's answers to questions, or try to change the patient's interpretation of the situation by "putting words into the patient's mouth"
- **Demand an explanation** – Do not ask "why" questions in an accusing tone
- **Give advice** – Only the physician advises
- **Demand an immediate response** – Allow the patient sufficient time for silent reflection before responding
- **Disinterested body language** – Do not appear distracted or make the patient feel inconsequential by impatient motions, bored posture, or rolling your eyes
- **Minimize the patient's feelings** – Do not compare feelings and experiences
- **Negatively empower** – Do not help your patient to manipulate another person
- **Make false promises** – Never promise the patient that the doctor will definitely cure the condition, or make promises that cannot be kept
- **Play into stereotypes** – Racist, sexist, and religious prejudice must not influence your treatment of the patient
- **Deliberately mislead** – Always disclose upcoming treatments, tests, or procedures

Pre- and Post-Examination Instructions

Some radiographic exams require patients to follow specific pre-exam instructions to better visualize the anatomy of interest. For example, patients may be asked to be NPO (take nothing by mouth including gum and smoking) eight hours prior to the exam. Others may require a colon prep starting the day before the exam to rid the body of excess waste to better visualize internal structures. Other times, the patient may need to be sedated, and it is important the patient is NPO so the patient does not aspirate. If patients are taking a medication to help them relax, they must be informed of exact times for the medication to be effective. Also, if patients have been sedated, it is important that they have somebody drive them home. Technologists should also be sure to give patients important post-exam instructions. For example, after barium studies the patient will need

Copyright © Mometrix Media. You have been licensed one copy of this document for personal use only. Any other reproduction or redistribution is strictly prohibited. All rights reserved.
This content is provided for test preparation purposes only and does not imply an endorsement by Mometrix of any particular political, scientific, or religious point of view.

to drink a lot of liquids and take a mild laxative to prevent constipation. Patients should also be informed of how the results will be communicated to them (typically from the ordering physician's office).

MRI Procedures

MRI stands for magnetic resonance imaging and is a procedure that does not use ionizing radiation. Instead, it uses magnetic fields and computer software to produce an image. The dye gadolinium is used as a contrast medium for the procedure. MRI is particularly useful in imaging soft tissue. Because it does not used ionizing radiation, there are, in general, fewer risks associated with MRIs. However, because it uses magnetism, any metal objects in the room or on/in the patient can become sources of injury. Also, because an MRI must be conducted within a close distance to the patient, many people experience claustrophobia. It is sometimes necessary to medicate the patient so that they remain still long enough to get a quality image.

CT Procedures

CT stands for computed tomography and is a highly specific application of radiation and computer analysis that is used to get a detailed, three-dimensional image. Because the primary beam of radiation is highly collimated (restricted) and delivered in a helical (spiral) fashion using slip ring technology, it can be precisely targeted to the area of interest to provide a multi-layered image. An iodinated contrast medium allows for the visual differentiation of different tissues. In order to get the quality image necessary for diagnosis, it is very important that a patient remain still for a CT procedure. It is sometimes necessary to medicate the patient so that they remain still long enough to get a quality image.

Ultrasound Procedures

Ultrasound (or medical sonography) creates an image by recording the echo of sound waves as they bounce off the anatomy to which they are applied. It is primarily a non-invasive procedure that does not carry with it the risk of exposure to ionizing radiation. For this reason, it is the primary means of visualizing the fetus during pregnancy. It can, however, be used in invasive procedures such as biopsy, intravaginal imaging, transesophageal echocardiography. To improve imaging, water is sometimes consumed so that the full bladder acts to magnify the anatomy being imaged. This is particularly helpful in fetal imaging.

Nuclear Medicine Procedures

In nuclear medicine, instead of the patient being exposed to radiation externally, they are injected with a radioactive isotope. Once the body begins to emit gamma radiation, the image is captured by a scintillation camera and analyzed by a computer. Because of the potential danger in working with radioactive materials, only nuclear medicine technologists are authorized to inject the radioisotope. It is a procedure that is extensively regulated by the NRC (nuclear regulatory committee). A department must keep very accurate records and properly dispose of nuclear waste in order to maintain a license to practice nuclear medicine.

Mammography Procedures

Used to detect breast cancer, mammography uses tissue compression and low doses of radiation to image breast tissue. It has become a highly regulated area of radiography that requires additional training and continuing education. The Mammography Quality Control Standards Act (MQSA) of 1994 and American College of Radiology (ACR) regulations provide the guidelines for mammography use and interpretation. Because breast tissue can be difficult to image using mammography alone, ultrasound, nuclear medicine, and MRI combined with the use of a breast coil can help give more accurate results. A biopsy (surgical or needle) is used to confirm the presence of

Copyright © Mometrix Media. You have been licensed one copy of this document for personal use only. Any other reproduction or redistribution is strictly prohibited. All rights reserved.
This content is provided for test preparation purposes only and does not imply an endorsement by Mometrix of any particular political, scientific, or religious point of view.

cancer. Appropriate film-screen combinations are necessary to get the best image. A computer image does not provide enough detail for an accurate diagnosis.

Procedures for 12-Lead ECG

An ECG (electrocardiogram) measures the electric impulses of the heart and is an indication of blood flow and heart operation. When placing a 12-Lead ECG, the patient should be laying down and covered with a sheet to maintain their basic privacy rights. The skin should be clean, dry, and devoid of hair. To improve conductivity, gel is applied to the skin before placing the lead. The leads are distributed between the limbs and chest. Proper placement is important in obtaining good results. If not placed properly, artifacts can result, obscuring the actual reading.

Physical Assistance and Monitoring

Proper Technique for Falling with a Patient

Even with all necessary precautions properly observed while ambulating, the patient is still at risk for falling. A fall may result if the patient's legs give out from under him or if he were to lose consciousness while ambulating. If a sudden fall were to occur, it is important to protect the patient and yourself from harm.

- Support the patient using the gait belt and your free arm, and gently lower the patient to the floor or to a nearby chair, taking care to protect the patient's head.
- If the fall is uncontrolled as a result of loss of balance, focus on supporting the patient as much as possible while keeping yourself safe.
- Try to avoid tensing up prior to impact as this may cause additional injury.

Proper Body Mechanics to Prevent Personnel and/or Patient Injury

Because patients are often ill or physically impaired and equipment can be heavy or bulky, it is important that a radiographer understands the basics of proper body mechanics so as not to injure themselves or the patient when moving a load. The basics of body mechanics are the same whether the load is a person or piece of equipment. Personnel must assess if the load can be lifted alone, with mechanical help, or with the help of another person. When moving anything, it is important to maintain a wide stance with a straight back and lift with the knees. Keeping the load close to your body and being sure that there is nothing that will impede movement will assure proper transfer of the load. When transferring a patient to or from a wheelchair or bed, always check to see if the wheel locks are set. Finally, make sure you clearly explain to the patient what you are going to do so that they do not hinder the move.

Devices to Promote Patient Safety

Common devices to promote patient safety include:

- **Lifts**: Utilizing lifts, such as the Hoyer lift, to assist in moving and lifting patients reduces the risk of falls and injuries.
- **Assistive devices**: Various assistive devices, such as canes, walkers, wheelchairs, grabbers, reaching devices, and medication dispensers, help to prevent falls, facilitate mobility, and promote safety.
- **Alarms**: Many types of sensors with alarms are available, including floor mat sensors, chair sensors, seatbelt sensors, and movement sensors. Door alarms may sound when doors are opened to alert staff.

Copyright © Mometrix Media. You have been licensed one copy of this document for personal use only. Any other reproduction or redistribution is strictly prohibited. All rights reserved.
This content is provided for test preparation purposes only and does not imply an endorsement by Mometrix of any particular political, scientific, or religious point of view.

- **Wander management systems**: Systems such as *Wanderguard®* and *RoamAlert®* require the patient to wear a device (such as a bracelet) that contains a locator and may also have a door controller to automatically lock doors as the patient approaches them or to sound alarm if the patient passes through an open door.

Patient Health Support

Vascular Access Devices

Many patients in need of a radiographic procedure have their health compromised in one or more ways. When a patient's health is compromised, any number of instruments or devices can be employed for patient health support. One such item is the use of vascular access devices (VADs). These are semi-permanent devices that allow access to a patient's veins to administer fluids, electrolytes, nutrients, and medications without having to stick the vein every time. They are used in chronically ill patients. The three types of VADs are central venous catheter (implanted into a large vein, usually the superior vena cava), percutaneous central venous catheter (implanted under fluoroscopic conditions into the subclavian vein), and implanted infusion port (surgically implanted into the infraclavicular fossa). All types of VADs must be kept clean and observed for the presence of infection. Care should be taken when moving a patient to not disturb or irritate the implantation site.

Oxygen

Many patients in need of a radiographic procedure have their health compromised in one or more ways. They may be critically ill, be suffering from injuries, or have an undiagnosed disease. When a patient's health is compromised, any number of instruments or devices can be employed for patient health support. One such item is the use of oxygen. Oxygen is a basic need for the functioning of the body. Most radiological suites have it available through ports in the wall; otherwise it is available in portable tanks. It is given to a patient in a humidified form (so as not to dry and irritate the throat and lungs) through a nasal cannula, oxygen mask, or mechanical ventilator. Flames or sparks should not be used in the presence of oxygen because of the possibility of combustion.

Intravenous Devices

Many patients in need of a radiographic procedure have their health compromised in one or more ways. They may be critically ill, be suffering from injuries, or have an undiagnosed disease. When a patient's health is compromised, any number of instruments or devices can be employed for patient health support. One such item is the use of intravenous devices. Commonly referred to as IV's, they are used to administer fluids, electrolytes, nutrients, and medications directly into the patient's bloodstream. Today, most IV fluids are administered using an IV pump. A radiographer needs to understand the basics of IV pump operation. Because every pump can be different, refer to pump instructions or consult nursing staff. The patient's chart must always be consulted before restarting an IV pump or replacing an empty bag so that the proper prescription is maintained.

Nasogastric Tube

Many patients in need of a radiographic procedure have their health compromised in one or more ways. They may be critically ill, be suffering from injuries, or have an undiagnosed disease. When a patient's health is compromised, any number of instruments or devices can be employed for patient health support. One such item is a nasogastric (NG) tube. This is a tube that is inserted into the nose, down the nasopharynx, into the stomach and is used to add or remove fluid in the stomach. If a radiographer uses the tube to administer contrast medium, water-soluble iodinated contrast medium (never barium) should be used. Care should be taken when working with a patient that has an NG tube so as not to disturb it.

Copyright © Mometrix Media. You have been licensed one copy of this document for personal use only. Any other reproduction or redistribution is strictly prohibited. All rights reserved.
This content is provided for test preparation purposes only and does not imply an endorsement by Mometrix of any particular political, scientific, or religious point of view.

Urinary Bladder Catheter

Many patients in need of a radiographic procedure have their health compromised in one or more ways. They may be critically ill, be suffering from injuries, or have an undiagnosed disease. When a patient's health is compromised, any number of instruments or devices can be employed for patient health support. One such item is a urinary bladder catheter (also called a Foley catheter). Inserted into the urinary bladder and attached to a bag, it is used to drain the patient's bladder. Some radiographic procedures require a full bladder, and so the catheter must be clamped and then unclamped for pre and postvoid films. Care should be taken when working with a patient that has urinary bladder catheter so as not to disturb it.

Closed-Chest Drainage Systems

Many patients in need of a radiographic procedure have their health compromised in one or more ways. They may be critically ill, be suffering from injuries, or have an undiagnosed disease. When a patient's health is compromised, any number of instruments or devices can be employed for patient health support. One such item is a closed-chest drainage system. It is used to remove air or fluid from the chest cavity after surgery or trauma. It helps prevent problems such as infection or a collapsed lung. Care should be taken when working with a patient that has a closed-chest drainage system so as not to disturb it. If fluid levels markedly increase or become bloody, nursing staff should be immediately notified.

Ostomy

If a patient's health is compromised, and any number of instruments or devices can be employed for patient health support. One such item is the use of an ostomy. It is a surgically created opening that allows for the exit of feces, urine or air from the patient's body. The different types of ostomies are: colostomy/enterostomy (opening through the abdominal wall into the colon for the removal of feces), ureterostomy (a procedure that brings the ureter up to the stomach for the removal of urine), ileal loop/incontinent urinary diversion (surgical movement of the ilium of the small bowel to the stomach for the removal of urine), continent urinary diversion (surgically implanted internal pouch that acts as a reservoir for urine). Care should be taken when working with a patient that has any form of ostomy so as not to disturb it. If a contrast medium is necessary, water-soluble iodinated contrast medium (never barium) should be used.

Tracheostomy

Many patients in need of a radiographic procedure have their health compromised in one or more ways. They may be critically ill, be suffering from injuries, or have an undiagnosed disease. When a patient's health is compromised, any number of instruments or devices can be employed for patient health support. One such item is the use of a tracheostomy. This is a surgical opening (tracheotomy) made into the trachea to allow for air flow into the patient's lungs. Many patients with a tracheotomy also require suction and oxygen, so it is important that a radiographer understands the use of both and has it available for use when necessary. Care should be taken when working with a patient that has a tracheotomy so as not to disturb it.

Suction

Many patients in need of a radiographic procedure have their health compromised in one or more ways. They may be critically ill, be suffering from injuries, or have an undiagnosed disease. When a patient's health is compromised, any number of instruments or devices can be employed for patient health support. One such item is the use of suction. It is used to remove fluid, blood, or mucus from a patient's airway. Like oxygen, it usually available in most radiological suites through a port in the wall. A disposable catheter is used to collect and dispose of secretions. The radiographer should be

Copyright © Mometrix Media. You have been licensed one copy of this document for personal use only. Any other reproduction or redistribution is strictly prohibited. All rights reserved.
This content is provided for test preparation purposes only and does not imply an endorsement by Mometrix of any particular political, scientific, or religious point of view.

familiar with the use of suction in patients in case the need should arise (particularly in patients with a tracheotomy).

Patient Safety

It is important that all medical procedures are safe for the patient. The basics of patient safety for medical procedures are as follows:

- Be sure to properly identify the patient.
- Conduct patient needs assessment.
- Use proper body mechanics so as not to injure yourself or the patient.
- Use safety straps, side rails, and immobilization devices properly and when necessary.
- Be aware of the location of the patient when moving equipment.
- Properly label and store patient personal belongings.
- Document any patient injury or property loss/damage immediately.

Monitoring Patient's Health and Well-Being

Although a radiographer is not a nurse, it is important that they have an understanding of some of the basics of clinical nursing so that a consistent quality of care can be maintained during radiographic procedures. Many patients in need of a radiographic procedure have their health compromised in one or more ways. They may be critically ill, be suffering from injuries, or have an undiagnosed disease. Because a nurse cannot always accompany a patient during a radiographic procedure, the responsibility of routine monitoring of patients can fall to the radiographer. It is important that the radiographer can recognize the signs of failing health and knows how to respond to medical emergencies.

Monitoring Vital Signs and Other Patient Indicators During CT Scanning

The machinery used to perform CT often includes provisions for monitoring the patient's vital signs, such as blood pressure, heart rate, oral temperature, and oxygen saturation. The test can be more effective if these vital signs are kept within normal limits, and doctors can choose to discontinue testing if the vital signs vary from those normal limits in response to the contrast agent, the duration of the test, or other factors. Patients are usually requested not to eat or drink for at least 4 hours before testing, although this requirement may be waived in an emergency. Patients should also be informed about immobilization on a hard table, venipuncture, a salty taste in the mouth, redness of skin during dye injection, mild nausea, diarrhea, and allergic reaction or kidney failure, which occur only rarely. Some patients are given a sedative for relaxation and easing of claustrophobia.

Physical Signs and Symptoms to Monitor

Technologists should always monitor patients for any sign of reaction to contrast or any decline of health during a procedure. Specifically, has there been a change in the patient's level of consciousness? Is the patient alert enough to comprehend and answer questions asked? Are there any indications of hives or cyanosis when looking at the patient's skin? Is the patient's breathing of normal rate and rhythm? A patient's pulse ox can easily be monitored should the technologist find it necessary to check. Technologists should be aware of any seizures that the patient may experience. Blood pressure is yet another important vital sign to monitor along with heart rate to determine the severity of a reaction to contrast, when caring for trauma patients, or during routine monitoring of a patient during an exam. If intravenous contrast was used, check for any signs of extravasation.

Copyright © Mometrix Media. You have been licensed one copy of this document for personal use only. Any other reproduction or redistribution is strictly prohibited. All rights reserved.
This content is provided for test preparation purposes only and does not imply an endorsement by Mometrix of any particular political, scientific, or religious point of view.

Creating a Safe Workplace Environment

One should take an active role in creating a **safe workplace environment** and preventing accidents:

- Slips: Most slips occur when the floor is wet or lacks adequate traction. Common causes include spills (water, urine, soap), oily substances (leaking oil), loose rugs and mats, and excessive floor waxing. Slips are especially a risk during wet weather as people may track water or snow in from outside. Floors should be checked and kept clean and dry,
- Trips: Most trips occur when the foot encounters obstacles (wrinkled rugs, cables, cords, clutter), view/walkway is obstructed, or lighting is poor. Traffic areas should be kept clear of clutter and lighting checked. Uneven steps should have warning signs.
- Falls: Many falls result from slipping or tripping, but some occur from a height, such as from a ladder or stairs. Patients who are unstable should always be assisted when walking and assisted at an appropriate pace.

Importance of Fall Prevention

Patient falls are a considerable problem in the health care setting. Injuries resulting from a fall are considered to be a primary cause of morbidity in older adults. The loss of coordination and bone density as people age puts them at an increased risk for breaking bones after a fall; the resultant loss of independence may lead to a decline in health and eventual death. Yet falling is not a normal part of aging. Proper prevention can greatly decrease a patient's risk of falling. As a nurse aide, it is important to follow fall precautions to prevent patient falls within the hospital setting.

Safety for Bed-Bound Patients

Patients who are bedridden have a particularly high risk of falling. The following are necessary safety precautions for bed-bound patients:

- While the patient is in bed, make sure the side rails are up to prevent the patient from climbing out of bed.
- If necessary, a bed alarm may be placed in the bed to alert the nurse aide that the patient is attempting to get out of bed without assistance.
- The patient's call light should be placed within reach, as well as the patient's tray table and any other items the patient might need.
- Toileting should be offered at least every two hours, and the patient should be turned every two hours to prevent bedsores.

Precautions to Prevent Falls

There are a number of precautions that can be taken to prevent patient falls.

- The first step of prevention is identifying the needs of the patient.
- If the patient has been determined to be a fall risk, a sign should be placed on the door so the staff knows the patient has special mobility needs.
- While the patient is in bed, at least two side rails should be kept in the raised position to prevent the patient from falling out of bed.
- Prior to standing with assistance, patients should be allowed to sit or dangle at the side of the bed to prevent dizziness that may result from the change in position.
- The patient should also wear rubber-soled shoes or socks.

Copyright © Mometrix Media. You have been licensed one copy of this document for personal use only. Any other reproduction or redistribution is strictly prohibited. All rights reserved.
This content is provided for test preparation purposes only and does not imply an endorsement by Mometrix of any particular political, scientific, or religious point of view.

- The floor should be kept free of all hazards, including puddles of water and small rugs that can cause slipping.
- While the patient sits in or stands up from the chair or wheelchair, the brakes should be kept locked.

Proper Documentation of Routine Monitoring

Proper documentation must be performed to provide the best patient care possible during the exam. Documentation also provides pertinent information that may be reviewed by clinicians and staff when follow-up studies are to be performed. When injecting a patient with contrast during exams, it is important to document the contrast media, dose, and any reactions the patient experienced. Routine monitoring requires the technologist to check for any change in the patient's mental status or other important vitals. Many symptoms can be monitored just by looking at or speaking with the patient. If the patient is suddenly having difficulty breathing, sweating profusely, bleeding, developing hives, or having a hard time speaking because of laryngeal edema, these are all signs that he or she is having a reaction to the contrast.

Vitals Monitored During Sedation

Technologists must always monitor patients for any sudden change in health. During sedation even more attention must be given to make sure the patient is not reacting to any medication that has been given. Important vitals to monitor are body temperature, which should be between 98 °F and 99 °F. The patient's pulse should also be observed and should be between 60 and 100 beats per minute. Respiration should also be checked and be between 12 and 16 breaths per minute. The patient's blood pressure is another important vital sign that should be evaluated. If the diastolic number drops below 50, it is an indication that the patient is going into shock. If the same number rises above 90, then one can assume hypertension. If the patient is on oxygen, the typical range is between 2 and 5 liters per minute. Suction should always be available in case it is necessary to remove secretions from the patient's mouth or throat. A patient will be hooked up to an electrocardiogram (EKG) machine, and it is important to watch for any signs of cardiac arrest in addition to respiratory arrest.

Medical Emergencies

Patients who are hospitalized, seen in the emergency room, or treated on an outpatient basis should be monitored in case a medical emergency arises. All technicians and hospital personnel caring for patients should be trained in basic cardiac life support. In addition, the hospital should have an emergency response system and protocol in place that any technician and/or health care practitioner can initiate, which may involve a hospital emergency response team or protocol. Health care practitioners and technicians should be trained in the protocol and system to be put into effect if a medical emergency occurs when caring for or performing a diagnostic approach on a patient.

Management of Medical Emergencies

In most cases, if a patient is in critical condition, nursing or emergency staff will accompany a patient for a radiographic procedure. If a patient appears to be stable, however, nursing staff may not be immediately available and the radiographer may be called upon to react if an emergency arises. For this reason, the radiographer must be familiar with basic protocol in responding to common medical emergencies such as allergies, head injuries, shock, high/low blood sugar, nosebleed, seizures, cardiac arrest, and respiratory arrest. It may be necessary to initiate a life-saving procedure before nursing staff can respond or assist in the procedure once they do respond.

Copyright © Mometrix Media. You have been licensed one copy of this document for personal use only. Any other reproduction or redistribution is strictly prohibited. All rights reserved.
This content is provided for test preparation purposes only and does not imply an endorsement by Mometrix of any particular political, scientific, or religious point of view.

Allergic Reactions

An allergic reaction occurs when the body's acquired immune system has an adverse response to a substance (allergen). In order for the body to recognize the allergen, there is an initial exposure that does not cause a reaction, but sensitizes the body to the substance. It is a subsequent exposure to the allergen that then results in an allergic reaction (called an inflammatory response). The reaction can be a simple irritation caused by contact to the substance, a delayed allergic reaction, or an immediate allergic reaction. Some allergic reactions are serious and require immediate medical assistance. A severe allergic reaction has respiratory symptoms such as itchy eyes, runny nose, sneezing, wheezing, and difficulty breathing. A mild allergic reaction can cause skin redness, hives, or itching. Medical products that contain latex as well as the contrast media used in certain radiographic procedures can cause mild to severe allergic reactions in patients

Latex

Latex products can cause mild to sever allergic reactions in patients. The reaction can be to the proteins in the latex itself, or to the other chemicals added to latex in processing. There are three types of reactions that can occur when a person is sensitive to latex products:

- Irritant Contact Dermatitis – Mild skin irritation that is characterized by dry, itch areas. This is not considered a true allergic reaction.
- Allergic Contact Dermatitis – Also called delayed hypersensitivity. Usually occurs 24-48 hours after exposure. Causes a rash to oozing blisters.
- Latex Allergy – Also called immediate hypersensitivity. Occurs within minutes to hours after exposure. Reaction can be mild to serious.

Common medical equipment that could contain latex are disposable gloves, tourniquets, blood pressure cuffs, stethoscopes, IV tubing, oral and nasal airway tubing, enema tips, endotracheal tubes, syringes, electrode pads, catheters, wound drains, and injection ports.

Cardiopulminary Arrest

Cardiopulmonary arrest is a serious condition that occurs when there is a sudden stopping of blood and air flow within the body. Every radiographer must be trained in the "ABC's" (airway, breathing, circulation) of CPR and know how it differs depending on the age of the patient. If a patient appears to be going into cardiopulmonary arrest, stop the procedure immediately and call for help. Start CPR and proceed until the emergency team arrives. Don't simply wait until the emergency team arrives, doing nothing. Immediate treatment is necessary to save the patient's life.

Respiratory Arrest

Respiratory arrest is the failure of the lungs to fill with air. There are two types of respiratory arrest: acute and chronic. Acute respiratory arrest is caused by an airway obstruction, which requires the Heimlich maneuver to remove the obstruction or ineffective gas exchange in the lungs, which requires the use of positive pressure ventilation. Chronic respiratory arrest is due to the progress of a disease such as emphysema, bronchitis, or asthma and may require the use of ventilation or suction. It is important to recognize the difference between respiratory arrest (the patient stops breathing) and cardiopulminary arrest (there is no pulse as well as the cessation of breathing) so that the proper emergency procedure is followed.

Head Injuries

If a person has experienced any type of head injury, they should not be left alone. While they may initially seem stable, there is still a chance that they will need to vomit, and with this comes the possibility of choking on the vomitus (aspiration). If it is necessary to leave the room, make sure

Copyright © Mometrix Media. You have been licensed one copy of this document for personal use only. Any other reproduction or redistribution is strictly prohibited. All rights reserved.
This content is provided for test preparation purposes only and does not imply an endorsement by Mometrix of any particular political, scientific, or religious point of view.

that someone is there to watch them while you are gone. If they need to vomit, provide them with an adequate container (like a large basin or bedpan). If they are lying down, turn them on their left side to vomit (the right side increases likelihood of choking). An individual with a head injury may also go into shock. It is necessary for a radiographer to know the signs and symptoms of shock.

NOSEBLEED

If a patient has a nosebleed, they should sit up if possible, otherwise raise their head. Use gauze to soak up the blood (not tissue), and have the patient apply pressure to the nasal septum. Applying ice to the nose is effective in constricting the blood vessels and slowing the flow of blood. The patient should be supplied with a basin to spit blood into and water for rinsing out their mouth. Bleeding should stop within ten minutes. If it does not stop within ten minutes or gets worse, call for medical assistance.

SEIZURES

If a patient experiences a seizure during a radiographic procedure, immediately stop the procedure and have the patient lie down. Cushion their head so as to minimize potential injury. To avoid choking, the patient should be turned on their left side; have suction and oxygen available and ready to use, should the need arise. Contrary to popular belief, they should not be restrained nor should anything be placed between their teeth. Monitor and time the duration of the seizure. When it is over, be sure to check the patient's vital signs.

HYPOGLYCEMIA

The key to responding to hypoglycemia (low blood sugar) is recognizing the signs and symptoms. These are tremors, sweating, sudden tiredness, hunger, syncope (fainting or dizziness). If hypoglycemia is suspected, first determine if the patient is a diabetic. If a glucometer is available and the patient is not rapidly failing, their blood sugar levels can be tested to determine if, indeed, it is hypoglycemia. To combat hypoglycemia, the patient needs to be given something that is sugary to eat. Glucose gel can be placed on the inner check, otherwise, orange juice or hard candy work well too. It typically takes 15 minutes to get the blood sugar levels back up. Once the episode is over, the patient's vital signs should be checked.

SHOCK

Shock can be the result of many different types of conditions. Because it can sometimes be serious, it is necessary for a radiographer to be familiar with the different types of shock. The causes of the different types of shock are as follows:

- Hypovolemic Shock: Low blood volume as a result of vomiting, diarrhea, hemorrhage
- Systemic Shock: Collapse of circulatory system as a result of intense infection
- Neurogenic Shock: Failure of arterial resistance due to head/spinal injury or neurotransmitter failure
- Cardiogenic Shock: Failure of the heart to pump due to pulmonary emboli (blood clot), myocardial infarct (heart attack), or pericardial edema (fluid around the heart)
- Anaphylactic Shock: Severe allergic reaction due to bee stings, medication, peanuts, or any foreign substance to which the body has not been exposed and sensitized.
- Syncope: Emotional response reaction due to fear, pain, or any severely unpleasant event.

Shock can be the result of many different types of conditions. Because it can sometimes be serious, it is necessary for a radiographer to be familiar with signs and symptoms of shock. Even though the

Copyright © Mometrix Media. You have been licensed one copy of this document for personal use only. Any other reproduction or redistribution is strictly prohibited. All rights reserved.
This content is provided for test preparation purposes only and does not imply an endorsement by Mometrix of any particular political, scientific, or religious point of view.

different types of shock are caused by many different conditions, the signs and symptoms of shock are the same for all. They are as follows:

- Hypotension (low blood pressure)
- Tachycardia (pulse over 100 beats/minute)
- Skin that is cool, moist, and pale
- Increased rate of respiration
- Decrease in mental coherence
- Anxiety
- Thirst

If the radiographer notices any of the above signs and symptoms, they should stop the procedure immediately and call for help. The patient should be lowered to the ground with feet elevated. For the sake of the wellbeing of the patient, it is important to respond immediately. Recognizing that a patient is in shock, understanding how to call in a code, and knowing the location of the code cart are all important steps in saving a patient's life.

Infection Control

Bloodborne Pathogens

Bloodborne pathogens are microorganisms in the blood or other body fluids that can cause illness and disease in people. These microorganisms can be transmitted through contact with contaminated blood and body fluids. The majority of the population immediately refers to the HIV virus or AIDS when defining bloodborne pathogens. However, hepatitis B and C are much more common in the medical setting.

Exposure to Bloodborne Pathogens

A medical professional can be exposed to bloodborne pathogens by accidental puncture wounds from needles, scalpels, broken glass or razor blades. An individual can also be exposed if contaminated body fluids come into contact with an open wound on the skin. The hepatitis B virus can actually be transmitted indirectly when a medical professional touches dried or caked-on blood and then touches the eyes, nose, or mouth.

Cycle of Infection

The cycle of infection starts with the presence of a pathogen (a disease-causing organism) and an environment that allows it to grow and multiply. Aside from being able to grow and multiply, the conditions must allow it to be passed on (transmission) from one organism (host) to another. Transmission can be either direct or indirect. Direct transmission occurs when the infection is passed from one infected host to another. There are several different possible modes of indirect transmission. An object can become contaminated and a person becomes infected when they touch the contaminated object (called a fomite). A vector can be employed by the pathogen, infecting an intermediate host where it can multiply and develop before being passed on to a new host. The pathogen can become airborne before finding a new host to infect. In any mode of transmission, there must be a way for the pathogen to enter the new host and the host must be susceptible to the infection.

Reservoir

Medical professionals must understand all five components of the cycle of infection to prevent the spread of disease. All of these factors must be present for an infection to transpire. They are a

Copyright © Mometrix Media. You have been licensed one copy of this document for personal use only. Any other reproduction or redistribution is strictly prohibited. All rights reserved.
This content is provided for test preparation purposes only and does not imply an endorsement by Mometrix of any particular political, scientific, or religious point of view.

reservoir host, exit mode, method of transmission, route of entrance, and a susceptible host. The first aspect takes place when a microorganism (pathogen) latches onto a living host. This living host is referred to as a reservoir host and may be a human, an insect, or even an animal. A reservoir's body will offer the proper nourishment for the pathogen for it to live and/or proliferate. When humans serve as the reservoir hosts, they become carriers of the disease but are often oblivious that they have been infected and can easily transmit the disease to other people. When there is evidence of a disease in a reservoir host, one may be more aware of hand washing and other methods to prevent the spread of disease.

PORTAL OF EXIT

The second step that must take place for an infection to occur is that the reservoir host provides a portal of exit. This describes the method in which the microorganism leaves the reservoir host to continue on to infect another organism, known as the susceptible host. The most prevalent avenues for exiting the body are via the mouth, nose, blood, urine, vaginal or seminal fluid, feces, and even the eyes. Often the portal of exit is the exact same as the entrance portals, which is the fourth step in the cycle of infection.

METHOD OF TRANSMISSION

DROPLET MODE OF TRANSMISSION

Droplet (mucous) particles may be transmitted when the reservoir host sneezes or coughs. It is known that the reservoir host does not need to be in close proximity to the susceptible host as droplet particles can travel several feet in the air. Respiratory diseases such as influenza and tuberculosis may be transmitted via a direct airborne method when the susceptible host inhales the droplets of the infected person. These types of infections may sweep through a population rapidly, so it is important to practice proper techniques to prevent airborne transmission. This includes coughing or sneezing into a tissue when possible. If a tissue is not available, one should sneeze or cough into the crook of the elbow and then perform proper hand washing. Often, patients who have a respiratory infection are asked to wear a mask to prevent the spread of infected droplets.

DIRECT CONTACT MODE OF TRANSMISSION

Bloodborne transmission may occur by direct mode if blood from the infected reservoir host comes into contact with the susceptible host's mucous membranes or when the integrity of the skin is compromised. Healthcare workers must always practice universal precautions and utilize personal protective equipment (PPE) such as gloves, gowns, masks, eye protection, and face shields to prevent blood from reaching these mucous membranes or from getting into any cut in the skin. The most common bloodborne pathogens that may be transmitted in a healthcare setting are hepatitis B (HBV), hepatitis C (HCV), and the human immunodeficiency virus (HIV). Healthcare professionals should assume and treat all bodily fluids as if they are contaminated, and any PPE should be managed and disposed of properly. Another example of direct transmission is when a pregnant female passes on a sexually transmitted infection (STI) onto her baby via the placenta or during a vaginal delivery, such as gonorrhea, herpes, or syphilis.

AIRBORNE MODE OF TRANSMISSION

The spread of microorganisms can take place when particles are dispersed from the respiratory system of the reservoir host and inhaled by another individual. This is known as airborne transmission. An example of airborne transmission is inhaling droplets when an infected individual coughs or sneezes. It is known that people do not need to be located right next to each other as these droplets are capable of traveling several feet following a cough or sneeze. This is a common method in which influenza, tuberculosis, or even chickenpox is spread. People may also become ill after the inhalation of bacteria or fungi within water that is contaminated. One example of this type

Copyright © Mometrix Media. You have been licensed one copy of this document for personal use only. Any other reproduction or redistribution is strictly prohibited. All rights reserved.
This content is provided for test preparation purposes only and does not imply an endorsement by Mometrix of any particular political, scientific, or religious point of view.

of airborne infection is Legionnaires' disease. This is not spread from person to person but rather when somebody inhales water droplets that contain the bacteria. This is often heard of in contaminated water supplies such as in hotels, resorts, or air-conditioning systems of apartment complexes.

Vehicle-Borne Fomite Mode of Transmission

A fomite is referred to any inanimate object that can spread a pathogen from one person to the next. Common examples of fomites that aid in the transmission of disease are doorknobs, drinking fountains, water glasses, pens, toys, books, and shopping carts. With these examples, it is easy to see why schools or child-care centers can readily spread germs among individuals. Note that this transmission is carried out in an indirect fashion as body membranes do not need to touch each other. Examples of vehicle-borne fomites in the medical industry could be instruments used in clinical care settings such as tools used for surgical procedures or patient care. Other examples of a vehicle-borne fomite in the medical field could be blood, biopsy specimens, or organs and tissues used for transplants or grafting material.

Vector-Borne Mechanical or Biological Mode of Transmission

A vector-borne method of transmission occurs when pathogens are spread from one living organism to another. Vectors are commonly insects that act as couriers that transport bacteria and other common pathogens from one individual to the next. Examples of vectors are mosquitoes, flies, ticks, and fleas. Mosquitoes are known for spreading West Nile virus. Flies can mechanically transmit disease as they continuously land on food and people. Infected ticks are widely known for spreading Lyme disease when they bite a person. Another disease that ticks may spread is Rocky Mountain spotted fever, which may be deadly if not diagnosed correctly. Fleas are the culprits in transferring pathogens that allow people and animals to contract the plague. Mosquitoes, ticks, and fleas tend to fall under the biological mode of transmission as they tend to become infected because they feed on the blood of their hosts.

Portal of Entry

A portal of entrance is the fourth step that must take place for an infection to occur known as the cycle of infection. As the microorganism exits the reservoir host, it must have an entrance portal to infect the susceptible host. Examples of entrance portals are similar to exit routes and include any mucous membrane such as the nose, mouth, rectum, or vagina. These pathogens can also enter via the integumentary system when the skin is no longer intact. The eyes are yet another entrance portal, and conjunctivitis is a very contagious disease that is spread via this entrance method. Urinary tract infections are another common infection seen, especially in females. This occurs as bacteria from the rectum are transferred to the urethra because of the close proximity of these structures. It is important to practice proper hygiene whether it is wiping after using the toilet or hand washing to prevent the transfer of bacteria and other pathogens.

Susceptible Host

A susceptible host is the fifth and final component in the cycle of infection. A susceptible host is an individual that is unable to fight off an infection and will enable the cycle to continue when this individual passes the pathogen onto another person. There are many factors that determine whether the susceptible host will become infected. These may include the strength of the immune system, overall health, and level of nourishment. Age is another important factor as infants and the elderly are more susceptible to certain diseases. Hygiene practices as well as living conditions are yet another determining factor that may induce an infection. For example, perhaps the host employs great hand-washing techniques but is forced to wash with water that is contaminated while living in a house with rodents and insects. Sometimes the susceptible host, regardless of how

Copyright © Mometrix Media. You have been licensed one copy of this document for personal use only. Any other reproduction or redistribution is strictly prohibited. All rights reserved.
This content is provided for test preparation purposes only and does not imply an endorsement by Mometrix of any particular political, scientific, or religious point of view.

healthy he or she is, may be infected with a microorganism so potent that the host is unable to fight it off even with a strong immune system.

Aseptic and Sterile Techniques of Venipuncture

During the physical act of administering medication, the practitioner should be aware of the basic tenets of sterilization. The medication or contrast agent must be injected with consideration for power injectors, other comparable methods, extravasation and treatment, and use of an IV pump. Any adverse reactions to contrast dyes, latex, or sedation and the treatment required for such reactions should be analyzed and included in the patient's documentation. The practitioner should always adhere to aseptic techniques and should verify that the area is free of pathogenic microorganisms so that infection can be prevented, according to the standards and guidelines set forth by the medical facility in which the venipuncture is being performed. All medical facilities must meet certain health codes regarding asepsis.

Surgical Asepsis

In order to prevent or control the spread of infection, the cycle of infection must be broken. The cycle of infection refers to the conditions that allow infection to spread. These conditions (presence of pathogen, growth and reproduction, transmission to host, susceptibility of host) must all be present in order for an infection to exist. Surgical asepsis (also called sterile technique) is a strict process of keeping an area sterile by removing any microorganisms from objects in the environment. This is done with the use of an autoclave, gas sterilization, or chemical cleaning solution. The area is them kept sterile by protecting it from contamination with the use of sterile draping, masks, caps, gowns, and gloves. Surgical asepsis should be used any time a patient is cut open for a procedure, if there is damaged skin (burns, cuts), or if a medical device is being inserted into a patient.

There are basic principles that govern surgical asepsis. They are in place to help keep an environment sterile, thus preventing and controlling the spread of infection. The most important (and basic) principle is that sterile objects remain sterile only when they come into contact with other sterile objects. No matter how clean the object it comes into contact with is, if it is not sterile, it should be considered a contaminant. If you are not sure if an object is sterile, or if the object is out of your field of view, it should be treated as contaminated.

Disinfectants and Antiseptics

Disinfectants are used to kill possible pathogens. They are bactericidal corrosive compounds composed of chemicals. Some disinfectants are capable of killing viruses such as HIV and HBV. These are not used on humans to disinfect skin. A common disinfectant is bleach in a 1:10 dilution.

Antiseptics are chemical compounds that inhibit or prevent the growth of microorganism microbes usually applied externally. Antiseptics attempt to prevent sepsis but do not necessarily kill bacteria and viruses. Antiseptics are used on human skin. Common antiseptics include70% isopropyl alcohol, betadine, and benzalkonium chloride with isopropyl alcohol being the most commonly used. Betadine is used when a sterile draw is needed.

Equipment Disinfection

The majority of supplies utilized in clinical settings tend to be disposable, but for those that can be reused, they must be properly disinfected or sterilized prior to another procedure. There are different levels of disinfection, but high-level disinfection is used when the equipment used has possibly been exposed to human immunodeficiency virus (HIV), hepatitis B virus (HBV), or hepatitis C virus (HCV). The steps for proper disinfection are as follows: remove equipment from

Copyright © Mometrix Media. You have been licensed one copy of this document for personal use only. Any other reproduction or redistribution is strictly prohibited. All rights reserved.
This content is provided for test preparation purposes only and does not imply an endorsement by Mometrix of any particular political, scientific, or religious point of view.

the patient, remove any protective cover from the equipment, wipe off any excess fluid, rinse under water while using a soap containing a germicidal solution, immerse (when allowed) equipment into disinfecting agent for the suggested time (check equipment manufacturer for suggested disinfection solutions), rinse with water, and dry. Caution must be taken to allow enough time between patients for the equipment to be properly disinfected.

Equipment Sterilization

Equipment must be sterilized if it will be used during any procedure that requires a sterile field. Instruments that can be sterilized are typically stainless steel and hold up well to sterilization techniques to be used again. The most common method of sterilization for tools used in the medical industry is an autoclave. This method utilizes steam and pressure to rid the tools of any microorganisms that are present. Once a procedure has ended the tools must first be rinsed, sanitized, and dried per the department's protocols. Some tools must then be wrapped in a special paper that is porous enough for the moisture to reach the tools or placed in special pouches that may be placed in the autoclave. The autoclave typically has presets that can be chosen pertaining to the materials used. Once the cycle is finished, be sure to place the tools in a cool, dry place, and be cognizant of the expiration date as many will expire after 30 days.

Medical Asepsis

In order to prevent or control the spread of infection, the cycle of infection must be broken. The cycle of infection refers to the conditions that allow infection to spread. These conditions (presence of pathogen, growth and reproduction, transmission to host, susceptibility of host) must all be present in order for an infection to exist. Medical asepsis (also called clean or aseptic technique) refers to cleanliness practices in a non-sterile environment. The point is to remove as many pathogens as possible from the environment and prevent the spread of those that do exist. The biggest thing that can be done in medical asepsis is the washing of hands. The basic technique of hand washing is the use of warm water, antiseptic cleaner, the removal of jewelry, and specific cleaning of fingernails. Hands should be washed before and after contact with a patient, after contact with organic materials or contaminated equipment, after removing sterile or non-sterile gloves.

Sterile Technique

Method 1

The practitioner should scrub a selected area for 30 seconds with a sterile swab that is saturated in a 0.7% aqueous scrub solution of iodophor compound; any excess foam should be removed with another sterile swab. The iodophor complex solution should be applied with a sterile swab beginning at the intended venipuncture site and using gradually increasing concentric circles until an area 3 inches in diameter has been covered. The solution should be allowed to stand for 30 seconds before venipuncture is completed. If the practitioner cannot complete the venipuncture immediately after the 30-second waiting period, then the area should be covered with dry sterile gauze. If the arm is bent or the prepared site is touched by fingers or any other nonsterile object, the entire procedure for sterilization must be repeated.

Method 2

Another method of administering contrast agents requires scrubbing a selected area for 30 seconds with a sterile swab that is saturated in nonalcoholic, 15% aqueous soap or detergent solution so that any fat, oils, extra skin cells, dirt, and other debris can be cleaned away. The soap froth can be removed with another sterile swab saturated in 10% acetone in 70% isopropyl alcohol. The site should then be allowed to dry. A tincture of iodine can be applied with another sterile swab beginning at the venipuncture site and using gradually increasing concentric circles until an area 3

Copyright © Mometrix Media. You have been licensed one copy of this document for personal use only. Any other reproduction or redistribution is strictly prohibited. All rights reserved.
This content is provided for test preparation purposes only and does not imply an endorsement by Mometrix of any particular political, scientific, or religious point of view.

inches in diameter has been covered. The site should then be allowed to dry. The iodine can be removed with a sterile swab saturated in 10% acetone in 70% isopropyl alcohol, which should be allowed to dry. The prepared area should be covered with dry sterile gauze if the venipuncture is not completed immediately. If the arm is bent or the site is contaminated, the entire procedure must be repeated.

Method 3

For patients sensitive to iodine, the practitioner can directly apply 1 mL (an amount approximately the size of a penny) of One Step Gel to the venipuncture site. Held at an angle of approximately 30°, the sterile applicator can be used to scrub in a circular motion for 30 seconds until an area 1 inch in diameter directly over the venipuncture site has been covered. The same applicator can then be used, beginning at the intended venipuncture site and using gradually increasing concentric circles, to cover an area 3 inches in diameter. A second sterile applicator can be used to remove excess gel, beginning at the center of the 3-inch area and using gradually increasing concentric circles. The site should be allowed to dry according to the manufacturer's instructions. If the practitioner cannot complete the venipuncture immediately, the area should be covered with dry sterile gauze. If the arm is bent or the site is otherwise contaminated, the entire procedure must be repeated.

Method 4

Method 4 is the only method for sterilization of the intended injection site that does not require application in gradually increasing concentric circles from the intended venipuncture site. A solution of 2% chlorhexidine gluconate in 70% isopropyl alcohol should be prepared in advance. The practitioner should scrub the intended site of venipuncture with this solution, making repeated back-and-forth strokes across an area 2.5 inches by 2.5 inches for a minimum of 30 seconds. This repeated motion should ensure that the area is completely wet with the antiseptic. The area should be allowed to air dry for at least 30 seconds. If the practitioner cannot complete the venipuncture immediately, then the area should be covered with dry sterile gauze. If the arm is bent or the site is otherwise contaminated, the entire procedure must be repeated.

Universal/Standard Precautions for Prevention and Control of Infection

Universal (also called standard) precautions were developed in 1991 when, to help prevent and control the spread of infection, OSHA (Occupational Health Administration) and the CDC (Centers for Disease Control) mandated that every patient and specimen be treated as if it is contaminated. These precautions apply to all blood and bodily fluids (including peritoneal, amniotic, vaginal, seminal, cerebrospinal, synovial and saliva, pleural and pericardial fluids). Care should be taken when handling any of these fluids, or items contaminated with these fluids. Personal protective equipment (PPE), hand washing, and preventative measures should be employed.

Isolation and Infection Control Practices

There are isolation and infection control practices that should be completed with every radiographic procedure. They are as follows:

- Wash hands before and after each patient.
- Change pillowcase and clean the table surface between patients.
- Place a sheet on table surface to help keep it clean.
- Provide a denture cup for patient.
- Put the cassette in a pillowcase to keep it clean.
- Clean contaminated surfaces immediately.
- Clean equipment before reverse isolation procedures.

Copyright © Mometrix Media. You have been licensed one copy of this document for personal use only. Any other reproduction or redistribution is strictly prohibited. All rights reserved.
This content is provided for test preparation purposes only and does not imply an endorsement by Mometrix of any particular political, scientific, or religious point of view.

- Wear appropriate barrier dress (mask, gown, gloves).
- Properly dispose of protective gear and contaminated materials.

Safe Injection Practices

The Centers for Disease Control (CDC) recommends healthcare facilities practice the following guidelines to reduce the risk of exposure to patients and staff. First, aseptic protocols should always be followed during sterile procedures. If there is any question that the sterile field has been compromised, it is imperative to start over. Healthcare professionals must understand that syringes, needles, tubing, and so on are to be used on only one patient. A needle cannot be changed on a syringe after the syringe has already been used on another or even to draw up other medications for the same patient. All supplies used for an IV are to be properly discarded after being used on one patient. Medication and solutions should be dispensed to a patient from single-dose vials. If there is residual medication, it should not be given to another patient from the same single-dose ampule. For more information please refer to the CDC website https://www.cdc.gov.

Safe Handling of Contaminated Equipment and Surfaces

There are levels of disinfection for contaminated medical equipment and surfaces. These factors largely depend on equipment manufacturer guidelines and whether the supplies can be heat sterilized. High-level disinfection is one method that can be used for equipment that cannot be sterilized with heat, but it is not appropriate for surface disinfection. Regardless of which level necessary, all items are to be rinsed, sanitized, and then per the vendor's suggestions utilize only the disinfecting agents mentioned. Products used for high-level disinfection are considered to be sporicidal agents, are extremely virulent, and should also be rinsed with water and dried after the chemicals are used. Intermediate-level disinfection will kill tuberculosis but will not be effective at eliminating the bacterial spores. Low-level disinfection is used for surface areas and instruments such as stethoscopes, blood pressure cuffs, electrocardiogram (EKG) leads and wires, and so on that do not touch the mucous membranes of the patient.

Disposal of Biohazardous Materials

Biohazardous materials include anything that has been soiled with blood or other bodily fluids. They must be placed in special biohazard waste receptacles so that they can then be disposed of properly. Sharps must be placed in the designated sharps container. Radioactive material must be allowed to decay before being disposed of. None of these items are a part of the normal trash pick-up. In fact, facilities spend large sums of money on biohazardous waste disposal. Heavy fines are the result if not disposed of properly. Biohazardous waste disposal is regulated by the EPA (Environmental Protection Agency), OSHA (Occupational Health Administration), and NRC (Nuclear Regulatory Committee).

Prevention and Control of Infection

Droplet, Airborne, and Reverse Isolation Precautions

Droplet isolation precautions should be used when coming into contact with diseases that are spread by droplets (includes meningitis, Mycoplasma pneumonia, rubella, group A strep). Patients should be placed in private rooms. Masks and gloves must be worn when treating the infected patient, and gloves worn when coming into contact with every patient. Airborne isolation precautions should be used for tuberculosis, measles, and varicella. These are diseases that are spread by microscopic particles that must be filtered out of the air with special equipment. Patients must be completely isolated in negative pressure rooms. Contact precautions (gloves, gowns) must be employed and respiratory masks worn when in the infected patient's room. Reverse isolation precautions are designed to protect a patient from the healthcare worker. They are employed in

Copyright © Mometrix Media. You have been licensed one copy of this document for personal use only. Any other reproduction or redistribution is strictly prohibited. All rights reserved.
This content is provided for test preparation purposes only and does not imply an endorsement by Mometrix of any particular political, scientific, or religious point of view.

cases when a patient is immunocompromised (leukemia patient, organ transplant patient). These patients should be isolated in positive pressure rooms that keep outside air and contaminants away from them.

CONTACT ISOLATION PRECAUTIONS

Standard/Universal precaution measures should always be used when coming into contact with patients and bodily fluids. Certain diseases, however, require more stringent isolation precautions because of their highly contagious nature. Infections of MRSA, Salomonella, E. coli, hepatitis A, severe herpes simplex, lice, and scabies all require contact isolation precautions. These precautions require that gloves and gown always be used when entering the patient's room. Gloves must be changed when they come into contact with infectious material. Essentially, there should always be a barrier (gloves, mask, gown) between you and the patient, and the barrier material must be disposed of properly

Copyright © Mometrix Media. You have been licensed one copy of this document for personal use only. Any other reproduction or redistribution is strictly prohibited. All rights reserved.
This content is provided for test preparation purposes only and does not imply an endorsement by Mometrix of any particular political, scientific, or religious point of view.

Image Production

Basic Principles of Ultrasound and Equipment

Transducer

Transducer Component Improving the Propagation of Sound into the Body

A transducer is shaped similar to a cylinder and changes one form of energy into a different form. The matching layer is located in front of the transducer's active element (PZT). Gel along with the matching layer serves to improve the propagation of sound into the body as well as add extra protection to the PZT crystals. Because PZT has an impedance of nearly 20 times more than the impedance found in skin, there must be a matching layer for sound transmission. If there was no matching layer, the sound would be reflected back to the PZT and prevent an image from ever being created. To overcome this mismatch of impedances and allow for sound transmission to occur, the thickness of the matching layer is one-fourth of the wavelength of sound within the matching layer.

Parts

The transducer has five parts, a crystal, the matching layers, damping material, the transducer case, and the electric cable. The crystal converts the electrical voltage into sound energy to transmit and then reverses the sound energy into electrical energy when the sound beam returns or echoes back to the transducer. The matching layers lie before the transducer element and make the acoustic connection between the skin and the transducer. The damping material, such as rubber, acts as insulation and decreases extra vibrations. The transducer case houses the entire crystal, damping material, and insulation from interference with the electrical noise. The electrical cable contains the wires to conduct and transmit the electrical impulses from circuit source.

Effect of Increasing Frequency on the Wavelength

The definition of wavelength is the length of one cycle. Wavelength will be displayed in any unit of distance, but the usual range in diagnostic ultrasound imaging is 0.1 to 0.8 mm. Sonographers should know that the medium and the sound source are factors that determine the wavelength. Wavelength is not a control on the ultrasound system that a sonographer can change. Rather, wavelength changes when changing transducers that have a different frequency. As the frequency increases, the wavelength will become shorter. Wavelength and frequency are inversely related as long as the biologic tissue stays the same. In order to calculate the wavelength of a sound beam in soft tissue, the following formula can be used:

$$wavelength\ in\ soft\ tissue = \frac{1.54}{frequency}$$

Using this formula, users can also visualize the inverse relationship between the wavelength and frequency.

Backing Material

Ultrasound labs use transducers that contain backing material. The backing material (also referred to as the damping element) is used to optimize the axial resolution. This is accomplished by attaching a mix of epoxy resin and tungsten particles to the back of the active element or piezoelectric lead zirconate titanate (PZT) crystal. This will decrease the length of the pulse duration because it inhibits the amount of time that the crystal will vibrate. Short pulses increase the axial resolution and create higher quality images. Nonimaging probes do not contain backing

Copyright © Mometrix Media. You have been licensed one copy of this document for personal use only. Any other reproduction or redistribution is strictly prohibited. All rights reserved.
This content is provided for test preparation purposes only and does not imply an endorsement by Mometrix of any particular political, scientific, or religious point of view.

material. Using backing material will decrease the sensitivity of the transducer and create a wide bandwidth, and the result will be referred to as having a low quality factor. Continuous-wave Doppler and therapeutic ultrasound transducers are known as high-Q because they have a narrow bandwidth.

Steering Linear Sequential Transducers

The image that is created with a linear sequential-array transducer is in the shape of a rectangle because the pulses are sent straight out from the transducer in groups. Due to the beam formers of modern phased-array technology, these transducers can be steered. These transducers are electronically steered and produce an image that is in the shape of a parallelogram when steering is implemented. Sound beams are sent out from a small arrangement of active elements on the transducer face. These transducers will never create images that are wider than the footprint.

Thickness of the Matching Layer

The matching layer should be one-fourth of the wavelength of sound. This layer offers protection for the crystals because the matching layer is located in front of the active element. The matching layer is also used (along with ultrasound gel) to increase the transmission capabilities of vibrations from the PZT crystals and the tissue being interrogated. Impedance (a number that is calculated by multiplying the speed of sound by the density of the medium) influences the reflections produced as sound travels from one medium to another. The matching layer enables the ultrasound energy to make a smooth transition from the probe into the patient's body.

Focusing Linear Sequential-Array Transducers

Earlier versions of the linear sequential-array transducers used fixed-focus techniques. This meant that either a lens was placed in front of the crystals or the active element was molded into an arc shape. In these examples, the user could not adjust them. Today's linear sequential (switched)-array transducers are electronically focused using phased technology. This technology allows the PZT crystal to send out pulses at different times. Certain returning reflections are postponed so that they don't all return to the probe at the same time. This phasing allows for signals to be returned constantly, which allows focusing at all depths.

Use of Lead Zirconate Titanate in Transducers

The piezoelectric effect is the creation of voltage as the result of applied pressure to these piezoelectric substances. Some piezoelectric materials can be found naturally; however, lead zirconate titanate (PZT) is man-made and is the most commonly used material in transducers because it can readily be manufactured. PZT is often referred to as the active element or the crystal in an ultrasound transducer. PZT is created when a strong electrical current and heat are administered to the active element. This process creates an active element that is polarized. Depolarization can occur if the transducers are exposed to high temperatures, so sonographers should be aware that they cannot be sterilized because the crystals will lose their piezoelectric properties. The thickness of the active element should be half of the wavelength found in the active element.

Linear Sequential Probes

Curvilinear array transducers tend to create an image that appears to be sector or fan shaped. As the ultrasound beam diverges further into the body, the line density increases because there is a larger gap between every scan line. As a result of these gaps, the far field demonstrates lower lateral resolution. Linear sequential (switched) probes have a large footprint, and the shape of the image is a rectangle. The crystals in linear sequential transducers are arranged beside each other,

Copyright © Mometrix Media. You have been licensed one copy of this document for personal use only. Any other reproduction or redistribution is strictly prohibited. All rights reserved.
This content is provided for test preparation purposes only and does not imply an endorsement by Mometrix of any particular political, scientific, or religious point of view.

and the pulses sent into the body will move straight ahead. Because the scan lines are evenly spaced and parallel to each other, the line density in the near and far fields will be identical.

Convex-Array Transducer vs. Linear Sequential Probe

In order to obtain the largest possible field of view in both the near and far fields, a sonographer would want to choose a convex-array transducer. These probes are also known as curvilinear or curved-array transducers. The image display from a linear sequential probe is one that is in the shape of a rectangle because of the arrangement of the active elements. They form a straight line that directs the pulses in front, but the curved array is a sector shape that is blunted at the top. The bowed shape at the top of the image directly correlates with the curved shape of the transducer. Because these images do not form a sharp peak at the top, they tend to allow for a wider field of view in the near field as well as the far field.

PZT Crystals in a Phased Array

Transducers that offer phased-array technology are considered to be very advanced technology because they offer focusing in all planes and at all depths. Phase delays are implemented with phased-array technology. Every active element is connected to the ultrasound machine's electronic circuit component. The PZT crystals can be activated in groups to produce signals that have to be returned to the receiver. These groups of elements are excited at time intervals that are very close to the next group thus creating very small time delays.

Shape of Images Using a Linear Phased-Array Probe

When a sonographer selects a linear phased-array transducer, the shape will be a sector shape that narrows to a sharp point at the top (fan shaped) although the face of the probe is flat. The footprint of a linear phased-array transducer is quite small, which enables the user to scan between the ribs; however, numerous elements are squeezed together within its compact size. The number of active elements ranges from 100 to 300. The shape of the linear phased array differs from that of a convex phased array because the curvilinear probe produces an image that is sector shaped but at the top it has a curved portion that matches the arc of the transducer face.

Transducer Formats Used in Real-Time Imaging

Linear array is a format offering a rectangular image of an area. It is most useful in small parts of the anatomy and in vascular imaging. It may offer additional formatting in beam steering and in virtual format, offering the ability to look at a trapezoid image shape which will give a wider view of the area. The Vector format offers a trapezoid image shape as well and is often used in abdominal, gynecological, and obstetric exams. The sector image is pie shaped and can be used in cardiac or abdominal imaging. The curved array provides a large field of view helpful in abdominal or obstetrical imaging. Modern advances to equipment and the development of specific transducers and formats help imaging to be specific and accurate.

Linear Array Transducer

The linear array transducer provides the image in a rectangle. It is used when ultrasounding small parts and for vascular imaging. Some linear array transducers can be used for beam steering, giving the ability to guide the gray scale picture more accurately. A trapezoid image shape can be displayed as well from a linear array, making the visual format wider and better for attaining measurements. A vector transducer also gives a trapezoid image and is useful in gynecological, obstetrical, and abdominal examinations. The sector picture is pie shaped, lending itself to cardiac, transcranial, and obstetrical examinations. The curved array allows for a large field of vision and is more commonly used in obstetrics.

Copyright © Mometrix Media. You have been licensed one copy of this document for personal use only. Any other reproduction or redistribution is strictly prohibited. All rights reserved.
This content is provided for test preparation purposes only and does not imply an endorsement by Mometrix of any particular political, scientific, or religious point of view.

Focal Zone of a Sound Beam

The focal zone of an ultrasound beam is the section of the ultrasound beam that is surrounding the focus (focal point). Because the focal zone is a more generalized area than the actual focal point, it is located in the near and far zones of the ultrasound beam. In fact, the focal zone is divided equally so that half is within the near zone and half is located in the far zone. It is recognized that the diameter of the ultrasound wave is fairly narrow in the focal zone, so objects that are imaged are considered to be more reliable than objects visualized at other scanning depths. This is turn results in better resolution; however, keep in mind that the focal point is where the beam diameter is tapered the most, so the best resolution is located here.

Ultrasound Pulse Repetition Frequency

Pulse repetition frequency (PRF) is the number of ultrasonic pulses occurring in one second. This value is usually expressed in kilohertz (kHz). Doppler ultrasound scanners use pulsed wave systems. The major advantages of using a pulsed wave system is that it allows measurement of depth and that the sample volume can be adjusted by the operator. For these reasons, pulsed wave ultrasound is used to provide data for color flow images. A limitation of pulsed wave ultrasound is that the maximum Doppler frequency that can be accurately measured (without aliasing) is only one-half of the pulse repetition frequency.

Changing the Spatial Pulse Length by Changing the Scanning Depth

Spatial pulse length has units of distance and describes how long a pulse is from its beginning to the end. The normal value of the spatial pulse length in diagnostic ultrasound ranges from 0.1 to 1.0 mm. The pulse length depends on the sound source and the medium, but it cannot be adjusted by the ultrasound user. The scanning depth has no effect on the spatial pulse length. Operators should be aware that shorter pulse lengths produce images that are more truthful. Short pulse lengths are created when a decrease in the number of cycles is contained within the pulse. The wavelength is also determined by the sound source and the medium; therefore, if shorter wavelengths are present, then shorter pulses are created.

Duty Factor

Duty factor is the percentage or amount of time that a system is transmitting sound. The duty factor is calculated by the following equation:

$$duty\ factor = \frac{pulse\ duration}{pulse\ repetition\ period} \times 100$$

Duty factor is a calculation that has no units; rather, it will be expressed as a percentage. The ranges of duty factor for clinical imaging are from 0.002 to 0.005 or from 0.2% to 0.5%. These ranges of diagnostic ultrasound indicate that a small percentage of time is spent transmitting a pulse and a large percentage is used for listening. For continuous-wave systems, the duty factor is 1% or 100% because a signal is always being sent, but of course it cannot create an image because there are not any signals received. A system with a duty factor of 0% means that a transducer is not being used.

Effect of Increasing PFR on the Duty Factor

The duty factor is the percentage of time that a transducer is actively transmitting a signal. The pulse repetition frequency (PRF) is defined as the number of pulses sent into the body in one second. Duty factor and PRF are both affected by the imaging depth and will have a direct relationship with each other. The PRF is inversely related to the depth of the object being studied as is the duty factor. As the depth decreases, the PRF increases because new pulses are constantly being sent because the listening time is less. If the depth increases, the PRF decreases (as will the

Copyright © Mometrix Media. You have been licensed one copy of this document for personal use only. Any other reproduction or redistribution is strictly prohibited. All rights reserved.
This content is provided for test preparation purposes only and does not imply an endorsement by Mometrix of any particular political, scientific, or religious point of view.

duty factor) because there is more listening time, so the return time has to be greater. If the PRF increases, the duty factor also increases because the amount of time that the system is "on" or transmitting a pulse increases.

Penetration Depth and Frequency

Two main items influence the amount of attenuation that a sound wave will sustain. The depth or distance that sound travels in the body is the first component. If a sound beam travels a greater distance, this will result in greater attenuation. More attenuation equates to a decrease in intensity of the sound beam. The frequency of the wave is the second item that determines the amount of soft-tissue attenuation. There is more attenuation in sound beams that have a higher frequency; therefore, lower frequency sound will provide less attenuation. Attenuation is directly related to distance and frequency. In order to provide optimal diagnostic images, one should use the highest frequency waves possible and still be able to visualize them at the depth where they are located.

Axial Resolution

Resolution refers to how precisely an object is being portrayed during a scan. Axial resolution allows the ultrasound system to distinguish between two structures that are parallel to the ultrasound beam (located in front of each other). Axial resolution will determine how close two structures can be yet correctly be portrayed as two separate reflectors on the ultrasound display. Axial resolution is measured in distance, and the units are typically in millimeters. Image quality and factuality are represented with axial distances that are lower numbers. In diagnostic ultrasound, the measurements of axial resolution typically lie in the 0.1 to 1 mm range. Shorter pulses and brief pulse durations will enhance the axial resolution. Axial resolution is considered to be superior to lateral resolution because pulse lengths are shorter than the width of the beam. Axial resolution is also known as longitudinal, range, radial, and depth resolution.

Effect of Increasing Focus

Axial resolution identifies reflectors that are parallel to the ultrasound wave, and it is determined by the pulse length and duration of the pulse. If more focal zones are added, the pulse length will become longer, which can degrade the axial resolution. Shorter pulses demonstrate better axial resolution as does less ringing in the pulse. If the sonographer increases the number of focal zones, there will be better lateral resolution, however, because the width of the beam is narrow. It is important to note that if a sonographer wishes to maximize spatial resolution, this will incorporate axial and lateral resolution.

Boosting Axial Resolution

Pulses that are short will generate images with improved axial (longitudinal, range, radial, depth) resolution. Shorter pulses are established by using a transducer that offers a higher frequency, which will automatically result in shorter wavelengths. Diagnostic imaging transducers contain backing material that will limit the amount of ringing in a pulse. This is also a way to create a short pulse and improve axial resolution. Although images cannot be produced from therapeutic ultrasound or continuous wave Doppler for many reasons, one reason is that they do not incorporate backing material. As opposed to imaging transducers, they are considered to have a high quality (Q)-factor and narrow bandwidth.

Example

Explain how to calculate the axial resolution while examining structures in the body using a 3.5 MHz transducer with a pulse length of 6 mm.

Copyright © Mometrix Media. You have been licensed one copy of this document for personal use only. Any other reproduction or redistribution is strictly prohibited. All rights reserved.
This content is provided for test preparation purposes only and does not imply an endorsement by Mometrix of any particular political, scientific, or religious point of view.

The axial resolution will be equal to half of the spatial pulse length, and the following formula can be used to calculate it:

$$axial\ resolution = \frac{spatial\ pulse\ length}{2}$$

In this example, the pulse length is 6 mm:

$$axial\ resolution = \frac{6}{2} = 3\ mm$$

Depending on the available information, the axial resolution may also be calculated by the following formula:

$$axial\ resolution = \frac{wavelength \times number\ of\ cycles\ in\ the\ pulse}{2}$$

To determine the axial resolution in soft tissue:

$$axial\ resolution = \frac{0.77 \times number\ of\ cycles\ in\ the\ pulse}{frequency}$$

Remember: When the axial resolution is calculated to be a lower number, better image quality will be demonstrated because the pulses are short.

Lateral Resolution

Resolution refers to how precise an object is being portrayed during a scan. Lateral resolution allows a user to visualize two distinct reflectors when they are perpendicular to the sound beam and lying beside each other. This type of resolution will determine how close two structures can be to each other and still be visualized as two separate objects on the ultrasound display. The units of lateral resolution will be any form of a distance measurement. Values that are smaller will represent echoes that are more precise. The narrowest part of the beam (focus) is where the lateral resolution will be optimal. Lateral resolution is also known as angular, azimuthal, and transverse resolution.

Lateral Resolution

The lateral resolution tends to change with the depth of the ultrasound beam. However, the region of the sound beam in which the lateral resolution is the best is at the focus. At the focus, the beam is, of course, the narrowest. Lateral resolution refers to just how close two objects can be to each other while lying perpendicular to the sound beam where the system can determine that they are separate reflectors instead of one. At the focal point, the objects will be further away from each other than the diameter of the beam, so it is possible to discern two separate structures. Sonographers should be aware that lateral resolution is equal to the beam diameter and smaller values imply better lateral resolution. If the scan line density is increased, the lateral resolution will be enhanced. Values that are higher will reveal image quality with less detail.

Effect of Imaging Depth on the Frame Rate

The frame rate refers to the capability of an ultrasound system to produce multiple frames per second. Temporal resolution, which shows how precisely an object in motion, is portrayed from one second to the next and is decided by the frame rate. The frame rate depends on the imaging depth because a reflector that is deeper in the body will result in a longer time of flight to return to the transducer. A structure that is deeper in the body results in a lower frame rate, which tends to

Copyright © Mometrix Media. You have been licensed one copy of this document for personal use only. Any other reproduction or redistribution is strictly prohibited. All rights reserved.
This content is provided for test preparation purposes only and does not imply an endorsement by Mometrix of any particular political, scientific, or religious point of view.

degrade temporal resolution. If a structure is located more superficially or more shallow, the time of flight is shorter, which results in a higher frame rate and better temporal resolution. Depth can be controlled by the ultrasound user.

Elevational Resolution

Resolution refers to how precise an object is being portrayed during a scan. Elevational resolution takes into account the portion of the beam that is perpendicular to the ultrasound wave and is also referred to as the slice thickness. Slice thickness determines if the returning signals are actually located above or below the imaging plane because sometimes, they will look as if they are within the beam. Sonographers are aware that the ultrasound beam is not a uniform shape, but rather it varies with depth and takes the shape of an hourglass. Because of this shape, some echoes may be included in the return signal, but they are actually located either above or below the ultrasound beam. Blood vessels or cysts may appear as if they are filled in due to the wider slice thickness. This happens when tissues that surround the blood vessel or cyst are being included in the image being sent back to the display.

Using a Phased Array with a Defective Crystal

If a sonographer is using a convex phased-array transducer, the image will appear as a sector shape that is blunted at the top. If that probe has a defective element, the user will visualize a vertical band of dropout directly under the affected crystal. A convex (curvilinear) probe contains numerous (120–250) pieces of active elements arranged beside each other in a curved line. The PZT elements are activated in groups sending out beams that are straight ahead, but the arced shape creates beams that are sent out in various directions. Linear sequential arrays are always parallel to each other because of the flat shape of the probe. If a sonographer is using an annular phased-array transducer with one ring that is damaged, there will be a horizontal band of dropout across the ultrasound image.

Using a Transducer That Has Malfunctioned

If a sonographer is using a linear sequential (switched) array transducer with a defective piezoelectric crystal, there will be vertical dropout on the screen beneath the active element that has been affected. Recall that the image created by a linear sequential probe is in the shape of a rectangle. The pulses sent into the body are fired in groups at different times, but at various locations along the transducer's footprint. These groups of pulses that are transmitted are sent out in a linear fashion and spaced evenly from each other, so the only part of the image that is affected stems from the scan lines created by the piezoelectric crystal that has been damaged. If a sonographer is using a convex phased array transducer the image will appear as a sector shape that is blunted at the top. If this probe has a defective element, the user will visualize a vertical band of dropout directly under the affected crystal.

Using a Mechanical Transducer That Has a Faulty Crystal

If a sonographer is using a mechanical transducer, it should be known that there is only one active element used to create an image. The shape of an image formed by a mechanical transducer is a sector or fan-shaped image. The beam is steered mechanically and has fixed-beam focusing because this type of transducer only has one crystal; if the crystal is damaged the user will not see an image. In other words, the image, as a whole, is lost. Mechanical transducers have been replaced by more modern transducers in which multiple active elements arranged in either a straight or curved line to send out pulses into the body. In these transducers a defective element will create either a vertical (curvilinear or linear sequential) or horizontal (annular phased array) band of dropout.

Copyright © Mometrix Media. You have been licensed one copy of this document for personal use only. Any other reproduction or redistribution is strictly prohibited. All rights reserved.
This content is provided for test preparation purposes only and does not imply an endorsement by Mometrix of any particular political, scientific, or religious point of view.

Low-*Q* Transducers

Low-*Q*-factor transducers are used for diagnostic pulsed-wave ultrasound because they offer improved axial resolution. Low-*Q* transducers contain backing material that controls the amount of ringing that takes place. By restricting the amount of ringing, shorter pulses are created. Shorter pulses will designate better axial resolution and, therefore, improved image quality. The fact that the pulses are shorter with axial resolution means that the majority of the ultrasound beam's energy will dissipate after the first couple of oscillations. Another advantage of low-*Q* transducers is their ability to offer multiple frequencies because of their wide bandwidth. Axial resolution offers the most accurate image in modern transducers and imaging systems. Recall that the accuracy of axial resolution is not affected by the depth of the image whereas elevational and lateral resolution is affected.

Bandwidth and *Q*-Factor of Nonimaging and Imaging Transducers

Nonimaging transducers are not capable of producing an ultrasound image. Examples of nonimaging transducers are continuous-wave Doppler that can be used to determine blood flow. Therapeutic ultrasound is another application that doesn't provide an image during use. These transducers do not contain backing material; therefore, they create long pulses. Long pulses, in this situation, refer to the length of the pulse as well as the amount of time that the crystal is excited. The lack of backing material also allows smaller reflectors to be converted more easily into electrical signals as they return to the transducer. Nonimaging transducers are considered to have a high *Q*-factor (quality factor), because the bandwidth tends to be narrow. Imaging transducers contain a layer of backing material. This is used to create short pulses by inhibiting the amount of time the piezoelectric crystals are vibrating. Remember that short pulses create diagnostic-quality images, but the layer of backing material tends to lessen the sensitivity. Probes that are capable of producing diagnostic-quality exams are referred to as low *Q*-factor and have a wide bandwidth.

Relationship Between Electric Frequency and Acoustic Frequency

The frequency of ultrasound transducers relies on how the active element is activated. These can either be determined by continuous- or pulsed-wave principles. Pulsed-wave ultrasound will send short electrical impulses that travel from the system to excite the piezoelectric lead zirconate titanate (PZT) element in the probe. In contrast, ultrasound transducers that are considered to be continuous wave tend to steadily induce an electrical impulse that activates the probe's active element. The following equation can be used to formulate the frequency:

$$electrical\ frequency = acoustic\ frequency.$$

In the above example, if the voltage is 12 MHz, this is the electrical frequency. Therefore, the frequency of the sound beam would also be equal to 12 MHz.

Pressure and Ultrasound Waves

Pressure is an acoustic variable that helps determine which types of waves are ultrasound waves. Pressure is the amount of force within a particular area, and it can be measured in units of pascals. Pressure is directly related to intensity; therefore, if the pressure increases so will the intensity. Ultrasound is a longitudinal wave that must travel through a material in order to propagate because it is unable to travel in a vacuum. Ultrasound waves are created when an object in motion oscillates. These vibrations produce a difference in pressure or density. Compressions occur when there is an increase in pressure or density, and rarefactions take place when there is a decrease in pressure or density. Pressure energy is synonymous with potential energy in the body, and it is the principal type of energy that is present in the cardiovascular system as blood is being pumped from the heart into the blood vessels.

Copyright © Mometrix Media. You have been licensed one copy of this document for personal use only. Any other reproduction or redistribution is strictly prohibited. All rights reserved.
This content is provided for test preparation purposes only and does not imply an endorsement by Mometrix of any particular political, scientific, or religious point of view.

B-Mode Image

Recall that B-mode imaging is also referred to as brightness mode imaging. This refers to a series of dots that are processed by the machine in which the amplitude of the reflector corresponds to a white or gray dot on the image display. The x-axis is the horizontal axis, which correlates to the depth of the reflector signal that is being returned to the probe. This information is determined by the time of flight. In soft tissue, the depth can be calculated with precision when the time of flight is known. The 13-microsecond rule also applies when the ultrasound beam travels in soft tissue. It is known that it takes 13 μs for sound to travel 1 cm. If the time of flight is 26 μs, the depth of the object being imaged is 2 cm.

Real-Time or Gray-Scale Imaging

The most basic form of real-time or gray-scale imaging is known as brightness mode. This method is more commonly referred to as B-mode imaging. B-mode was the first gray-scale imaging method available. During B-mode, pulses are sent into the body and when the signal returns it appears as a dot on the screen. The amplitude or strength of the reflectors will be visualized as dots. Higher amplitudes will appear as bright-white areas on the screen. The areas that return weaker signals will be discerned as a gray dot on the image display. Even when color mode is used, the underlying image showing the actual anatomy of the patient is represented by gray-scale imaging.

M-Mode

M-mode ultrasound refers to motion mode. The data acquired are considered to be axial with regard to the location of the transducer because these data are collected along one line of sight within the ultrasound beam. M-mode also offers information pertaining to time, which is represented by the x-axis. As the reflectors move across the screen, they are visualized as the activity is taking place at that specific instant. As the structures move from left to right across the screen, they may shift up or down. This demonstrates whether the object is moving toward or away from the transducer. The y-axis represents the depth of the objects that are in the path of the ultrasound beam. Amplitude is also reflected because some objects will have stronger returning signals than others.

Interpreting the Display from M-Mode

Motion mode (M-mode) is represented by an x-axis and a y-axis. The x-axis is the horizontal portion of the display that equates to time. The vertical axis is the y-axis, and it correlates to the depth of the reflectors. The go-return time is a way to calculate the depth of the reflector. A higher go-return time correlates to structures that are deeper in the body, and smaller time-of-flight values are the result of signals that are shallower. Moving from right to left, if the tracing moves up, this indicates that the object is closer to the probe. A line that is moving down means that it is moving away from the probe. If the line is a horizontal tracing, it means that the reflector is not in motion.

Disadvantage of Pulsed-Wave Doppler

One major disadvantage of pulsed-wave Doppler is the inability to accurately measure high-velocity blood flow. When incorrectly portrayed, high-velocity flow will appear to wrap around the spectral window and look as if it is moving in the wrong direction. This phenomenon is known as aliasing and is a misrepresentation that is frequently seen with pulsed-wave Doppler. While using pulsed-wave Doppler, the sonographer should be aware of steps to take in order to eliminate aliasing. These include setting the scale as high as possible, adjusting the baseline, selecting a lower frequency, and finding a window that will be in a more shallow location. Also, it is important to note that aliasing will never take place when using continuous-wave Doppler.

Copyright © Mometrix Media. You have been licensed one copy of this document for personal use only. Any other reproduction or redistribution is strictly prohibited. All rights reserved.
This content is provided for test preparation purposes only and does not imply an endorsement by Mometrix of any particular political, scientific, or religious point of view.

SCAN LINE REQUIREMENTS

The velocity scale (also referred to as the pulse repetition frequency [PRF]) is a control that sonographers are familiar with during color and pulsed-wave Doppler imaging. The PRF controls how rapidly data sampling takes place, and it will allow the ultrasound system to increase or decrease the Doppler shifts that are displayed. A high PRF enables more sampling to take place because there is less listening time between the pulses that are being transmitted into the body. It is important to have the PRF set correctly during both modalities so that aliasing does not occur. Color Doppler enables ultrasound users to determine the direction of flow when present, and it requires 8 pulses/scan line. Spectral analysis allows operators to measure velocities as well as provide information about the direction and presence of flow, but it requires more effort at 256 pulses/scan line.

COLOR DOPPLER WITH ANEMIC PATIENT

If a patient is anemic, he or she has a lower than normal amount of red blood cells circulating in the blood. Some patients may be anemic because they do not have enough hemoglobin in their blood. Hemoglobin is a protein that contains iron, which transports oxygen from the lungs to all of the body's cells. A patient with anemia will still have a sufficient amount of red blood cells in their circulatory system to be able to successfully perform a color Doppler exam. For diagnostic ultrasound imaging, the main reflectors that provide information pertaining to Doppler frequencies are the red blood cells. Because the blood is constantly being transported throughout the heart and blood vessels, even a patient that is considered to be anemic will have a sufficient amount of red blood cells for a successful Doppler exam.

COLOR DOPPLER ANGLE AND FLOW

If color is not displayed within a vessel after turning on color Doppler, the sonographer should immediately consider the angle of the incident beam with regard to the flow angle. If the incident beam is 90 degrees to the blood vessel being interrogated, then the color will not be visualized. According to the Doppler equation, the cosine of 90 is zero; therefore, no color can be visualized. The next thing that a sonographer can do in order to improve visualization of color Doppler is to angle the color box so that the incident beam is not 90 degrees. Yet another adjustment that an ultrasound user can make is to increase the scale and the color gain in order to increase the amount of blood visualized in the vessel.

COLOR FLOW IMAGING APPLICATIONS

Red blood cells make up roughly 45% of the blood in the human circulatory system. Red blood cells supply all of the cells in the body with the necessary oxygen so they can carry out their functions. If color Doppler is applied, the reflections that are visualized are the movement of the red blood cells within the heart and blood vessels. In low-flow states, the moving blood may even be seen without turning on color Doppler. It is imperative that the user pays close attention to the color map because it will provide information pertaining to the direction the blood is moving and the velocity. If red is displayed at the top of the color map, it represents blood moving toward the transducer. If blue is on the bottom, it represents blood traveling in a direction away from the transducer.

ADJUSTING PACKET SIZE

When sonographers are using color Doppler and are trying to decide if the packet size should be adjusted, he or she should be aware that the packet size can, in fact, be changed. The velocity of blood flow can be truer to form if the packet size is increased, but the frame rate may suffer as a result. Color Doppler requires every scan line to be pulsed more than once. The packet size (ensemble length or shots per line) represents these numerous pulses sent out for each scan line.

Copyright © Mometrix Media. You have been licensed one copy of this document for personal use only. Any other reproduction or redistribution is strictly prohibited. All rights reserved.
This content is provided for test preparation purposes only and does not imply an endorsement by Mometrix of any particular political, scientific, or religious point of view.

The level of the packet size can be raised when trying to image smaller vessels that are within the venous system because the ultrasound machine will be able to detect low-flow states more readily.

Pulsed-Wave (Spectral) Doppler

Pulsed-wave Doppler is used to calculate the velocity of red blood cells that are moving within various blood vessels. From these calculations, the peak systole, end diastole, pulsatility index, and resistive index can be calculated; they provide useful information to clinicians pertaining to any pathology. The ultrasound user can choose the exact location where the measurements should be taken by placing the gate within the lumen of the vessel. The gate size can be adjusted if necessary, to get a more precise measurement. Aliasing may be a concern when using pulsed-wave Doppler, so the user may need to adjust the scale or depth of the anatomical structure being imaged, switch to a transducer with a lower frequency, or switch to continuous-wave Doppler. If the velocities are too high to be accurately measured, then the user should switch to continuous-wave Doppler to obtain the maximum velocity.

Obtaining Measurements of Blood Flow Velocity

Spectral analysis is the technique used during pulsed Doppler to provide information pertaining to the various velocities obtained in the blood vessel or organ. Blood doesn't travel in the same direction or speed even when contained in the same sample volume. The spectral analysis window will allow clinicians to examine how the frequency shifts are dispersed within the Doppler signal. Two types of spectral analysis that are used are the fast Fourier transform (FFT) and autocorrelation. FFT is the method used to operate the spectral analysis during pulsed-wave and continuous-wave Doppler. This method can determine if the flow pattern is turbulent or if it is normal (laminar) flow. Autocorrelation is only used during color Doppler, but it is faster than the FFT method. The gate can be moved until it is where the user wants to perform a spectral analysis. The size of the gate can be changed so that it is only within the vessel that is being examined. For example, if one is sampling the carotid artery, but the spectral display is also showing venous flow, the technician will reduce the size of the gate and reposition it so only the artery is being interrogated.

Advantages and Disadvantages of Power Doppler

Power Doppler (also referred to as energy mode or color angio) is a form of color Doppler that does not display the speed of blood flow or any directional information. Rather, it only determines that a Doppler shift has taken place and shows the amplitude of the moving blood. If there are more red blood cells in one area, the signals will be brighter. Vessels represented with power Doppler will all be identical colors on the display. Advantages of power Doppler include the fact that aliasing does not occur because the speed and direction of blood flow is not applicable. Power Doppler picks up blood flow in smaller vessels and slow blood flow because of its increase in sensitivity. There is an increase in sensitivity because power Doppler is not altered by the Doppler angle. A disadvantage of power Doppler is that, due to the increased sensitivity, flash artifact may be visualized when the patient moves or breathes. Power Doppler does not evaluate the direction or velocity of blood flow. When compared to color Doppler, the temporal resolution is greatly reduced.

Ultrasound Phantoms

A phantom is a structure that contains one or more substitutes for human tissue. It is used to simulate ultrasound interactions in various parts the human body. Phantoms are used to perform numerous tasks on ultrasound equipment such as testing sensitivity, contrast resolution, axial resolution, and lateral resolution. This also includes teaching ultrasound techniques, and servicing the equipment. The most important aspect of a phantom used for ultrasound is that the speed of sound in the test object (phantom) is equal to the speed of sound in the target human tissue.

Copyright © Mometrix Media. You have been licensed one copy of this document for personal use only. Any other reproduction or redistribution is strictly prohibited. All rights reserved.
This content is provided for test preparation purposes only and does not imply an endorsement by Mometrix of any particular political, scientific, or religious point of view.

Relationship of Density and Propagation Speed of Sound

Propagation speed describes how fast an ultrasound wave can travel through the body. The propagation speed depends on the medium; ultrasound waves cannot travel in a vacuum, so they must travel through tissue in order to propagate. The speed is associated with the density and the stiffness of the tissue being evaluated. The concentration of tissue within a volumetric area is referred to as the density. Density can be thought of as the weight of the medium, and tissues within the body have varying densities. There is an inverse relationship between the density of the medium and the propagation speed. This means that the denser a medium is, the slower the ultrasound wave will travel through the tissue. The speed of sound in soft tissue is about 1540 m/s.

Effect of the Stiffness of a Medium

The speed of sound is affected by the density and stiffness of a medium as it passes through a particular substance. Stiffness is also referred to as bulk modulus, and it determines how a particular medium will react when pressure is applied to it. As the stiffness of a medium increases, the velocity of sound waves moving through that material also increases. When the bulk modulus of the medium decreases; the speed of sound will be slower. Conversely, if the density increases, the speed of sound in the tissue tends to be faster. Stiffness can be thought of as a resistance to compress, and these substances are typically objects that are denser. There is a direct relationship between the stiffness of an object and the speed of propagation.

Calculating the Depth of an Object

Ultrasound systems can determine the depth of an object by calculating the time of flight. This time refers to the transducer sending out a pulse, and once the reflector has been identified, the signal is returned back to the transducer. The round trip of the pulse is calculated by the range equation and allows for a very precise calculation: $d = 1ct$, where d is the depth, c is the speed of sound in soft tissue, and t is the time of flight. The ultrasound system is designed to recognize the speed of sound in soft issue as 1540 m/s (1.54 mm/μs). Sonographers should realize that the time of flight is directly associated with the depth. If an object being imaged is shallow, the time of flight is short. On the other hand, if the reflector is deeper, the time of flight is greater.

Identical Impedance and Normal Incidence

Recall that incident intensity is the intensity of a sound beam prior to coming into contact with a boundary. The transmitted intensity is the forward propagation of the intensity of the incident beam after hitting that boundary. Normal incidence is when the incident sound beam comes into contact with the boundary at a 90-degree angle. Note that a reflection will only occur if the two types of tissue have different impedances; otherwise, transmission occurs. During diagnostic imaging, there is very little difference in the impedance of soft-tissue boundaries; therefore, greater than 99% of the incident beam will be transmitted. To summarize, with normal incidence (90 degrees) and identical impedance of the media, all of the incident beam's intensity will be transmitted. Keep in mind that the incident and transmitted intensities must always equal 100%.

Cleaning Up Low-Level Reflections in the Near Field

When a sonographer notices low-level reflections within the near field of a well-distended urinary bladder and would like to clean them up, he or she may do so using the reject control on the ultrasound system. On some machines, this may be known as rejection, threshold, or suppression, and it can be used to exclude weakened echoes from appearing on the ultrasound screen. Electronic noise produces low-level reflections, so the reject control can be used to reduce this noise. Because every echo must have a set minimum amplitude in order to be displayed, this control determines what that value is so that the signals are not processed, thus eliminating the noise.

Copyright © Mometrix Media. You have been licensed one copy of this document for personal use only. Any other reproduction or redistribution is strictly prohibited. All rights reserved.
This content is provided for test preparation purposes only and does not imply an endorsement by Mometrix of any particular political, scientific, or religious point of view.

Effect of Increasing Density and Speed on Impedance

Impedance can be defined as the obstruction of the transmission of sound as it attempts to move through tissue. Impedance is the product of a medium's density and propagation speed of the medium, so if the density and speed increase, impedance will also increase. Acoustic impedance is a calculation that has an impact on the amount of reflection that occurs. If two tissue types have the same impedance, then all of the sound will be transmitted. If two tissue types have vastly different impedances, then the majority of the sound will be reflected. For example, sonographers cannot easily image an adult brain because very little sound will be transmitted through the skull. If a sonographer is imaging a soft tissue and bone interface, almost all of the sound will be reflected from the bone. In the example of an ultrasound of the adult brain, a low-frequency transducer would have to be used, which will provide images with poor detail.

Measuring Intensity Changes

Decibels (dB) are a logarithmic ratio between the amplitude, power, and intensity of the ultrasound beam. Decibels are calculated by dividing the most recent intensity measurement by the original intensity measurement. A positive change in decibels indicates that the intensity of the wave is becoming larger or increasing. When there is a +3 dB change, the intensity of the wave is twice as large. A +10 dB change indicates that the intensity is 10 times greater. A negative decibel change represents a signal that is becoming weaker or decreasing. In the example above, a –3 dB indicates a reduction of the signal by half of the original intensity. If there is a change of –10 dB, it represents a reduction of the original beam by one-tenth.

Sources of Artifacts

Sources of artifacts:

- Acoustic interactions within tissues
- Instrumental factors (failures)
- Implanted devices
- Operator induced

Most tissue artifacts are well understood and taken into account for diagnoses.

Rate of Attenuation in Bone, Lung, and Soft Tissue

Attenuation refers to the weakening of sound waves traveling through tissue. As sound travels, there will be a reduction in the intensity of the wave. When comparing the attenuation rates of tissue within the body, soft tissue will fall in the middle range. Examples of soft tissue are structures such as the liver, spleen, brain, and kidneys. The media that have the lowest rate of attenuation are bodily fluids such urine, amniotic fluid in pregnant women, and blood. Water has no attenuation when examined with low-frequency transducers. Bone tends to absorb a large portion of the ultrasound beam, which allows for a high rate of attenuation when compared to soft tissue. In the lungs, air tends to allow for the absorption of the sound wave; therefore, air is considered to have the highest attenuation rate.

Components of Attenuation

Recall that as sound beams pass through the body, the intensity is diminished (as are the amplitude and power). Three components contribute to the attenuation of a sound beam: reflection, scattering, and absorption. Reflection occurs if a part of the sound beam is sent back toward the transducer. There are two types of reflection: specular and diffuse. Specular reflection takes place when there is a smooth boundary. This portion of the beam, however, does not return directly back to the transducer, but at an angle. Diffuse reflections take place at a boundary that is not smooth

Copyright © Mometrix Media. You have been licensed one copy of this document for personal use only. Any other reproduction or redistribution is strictly prohibited. All rights reserved.
This content is provided for test preparation purposes only and does not imply an endorsement by Mometrix of any particular political, scientific, or religious point of view.

and tends to reflect in various directions known as backscatter. Scattering is the second component of attenuation and occurs when the energy tends to travel in many directions. One cannot predict where scattering will take place. Absorption is the third component of attenuation, and this is when the energy of the ultrasound wave is converted to heat.

Relationship Between Scattering and Frequency

The correlation between scattering and frequency is a direct relationship. Lower frequency sound waves tend to result in less scatter than higher frequency waves. Higher frequency waves will scatter more than those waves that have a lower frequency. Scattering is a process that can be described as either a random or an organized modification of the direction of the sound beam. An example of organized scatter is Rayleigh scattering. This process tends to alter the direction of the sound wave 360 degrees. Rayleigh scattering also has a direct relationship with the frequency of the sound beam and can be represented by taking the frequency to the fourth power. For example, if the frequency triples, the Rayleigh scattering can be calculated by taking the frequency to the fourth power: $(3 \times 3 \times 3 \times 3) = 81$.

Half-Value Layer Thickness

The half-value layer thickness refers to how far sound is transmitted in order for the intensity of the wave to be reduced to half of the original intensity. The half-value layer is also known as the penetration depth or half boundary layer and describes attenuation. It can be calculated by the following formula:

$$Penetration\ depth = \frac{3}{attenuation\ coefficient}$$

Intensity is measured in decibels, so it can also be thought of as the distance that ultrasound will travel in tissue to reduce the original intensity by 3 dB. For diagnostic imaging, the range of the half-value layer is 0.25 to 1.0 cm. This thickness depends on the of the sound as well as the medium it is transmitted in. Half-value layers tend to be smaller for sound traveling at a higher frequency and those tissues that have higher attenuation rates. The half-value layer is greater for lower frequency sound and tissues that have a lower attenuation rate.

Rayleigh Scattering

Recall that scattering is an erratic, unsystematic diversion of the ultrasound beam in multiple directions. Rayleigh scattering is just one type of scattering, but instead of being erratic, the sound wave is directed in 360 degrees in an organized manner. Rayleigh scattering takes place because the actual size of the target is much smaller than the wavelength of the ultrasound beam. For example, if a sonographer can visualize blood flow in hepatic vessels without color flow Doppler, it is due to Rayleigh scattering. The red blood cells are the target of the ultrasound system, but the image may be misinterpreted because without color flow, the vessels may appear as if they are clotted. If the user decreases the frequency, then the signal amplitude of what may appear as a clot in the hepatic vessels should be less apparent. Rayleigh scattering is proportional to the frequency to the fourth power.

Intensity Limits for Unfocused and Focused Ultrasound

During an exam, the sonographer must keep the range of output intensity (or the energy of the ultrasound beam) within an acceptable level to reduce the chances of bioeffects. During an ultrasound study, the sonographer must be aware of the output intensity (or energy) of the ultrasound beam in order to reduce the chances of bioeffects to the patient. This intensity is called the spatial peak temporal average (SPTA), and it is the most pertinent intensity with regard to

Copyright © Mometrix Media. You have been licensed one copy of this document for personal use only. Any other reproduction or redistribution is strictly prohibited. All rights reserved.
This content is provided for test preparation purposes only and does not imply an endorsement by Mometrix of any particular political, scientific, or religious point of view.

tissue heating. If an unfocused ultrasound beam is used, there must be a lower intensity limit set versus if a focused transducer is used. An unfocused beam is wider, and it allows more ultrasound energy to reach a greater cross-sectional area of tissue. Therefore, to compensate for the wide beam exposure to the patient, 100 mW/cm^2 is used for the intensity threshold of an unfocused beam. A focused beam intensity limit, which exposes less tissue to the energy of the ultrasound beam, is safely set at 1 W/cm^2 or 1,000 mW/cm^2.

Safely Making the Entire Image Darker

Sonographers should always keep the as low as reasonably achievable (ALARA) principle in mind during all diagnostic imaging exams. This principle is followed in order to reduce the possibility of bioeffects during an ultrasound exam. Two controls on the machine will make an entire image darker or brighter as the result of adjusting the knob. In this example, the entire image is too bright, and the user wants to darken it. The sonographer may want to decrease the amount of receiver gain in order to darken the image. However, this is not the best step to take in order to demonstrate knowledge of the ALARA principle. Receiver gain will allow an image to become darker (or brighter), but using this control has no effect on the exposure to the patient. If one needs to darken an image while lessening patient exposure, the user should decrease the output (acoustic) power. This will result in a lower patient exposure because the strength of the voltage applied to the PZT crystals is weaker.

Ultrasound Technique Impact on Patients

Ultrasound should only be used for clinical exams in which the benefits outweigh the risks. One risk during an exam is an elevation of temperature in tissues exposed to the ultrasound beam. The thermal index (TI) will be highest during an exam with a high-frequency, high-intensity beam. This heating depends on exposure time and temperature. Typically, the greatest increase in temperature is witnessed with spectral Doppler exams. Pulsed-wave Doppler requires more energy than B-mode or gray-scale imaging. Ideally, the TI should be 1.0 or less and the time should be minimized to prevent tissue heating. If the TI is 1.0, it means that there is a possibility that the temperature of tissue will increase by 1 degree. TI is expressed by the soft-tissue thermal index (TIS), bone thermal index (TIB), and cranial bone thermal index (TIC).

Ultrasound Application with Lowest Levels of Tissue Heating

It is no surprise that the lowest level of tissue heating occurs when the output intensity of the equipment being used is at its lowest numerical value. Generally, grayscale imaging is the method in which tissue heating will be the lowest. It is typically the highest when pulsed Doppler is being used. M-mode and color flow Doppler tend to fall in the middle of these intensities. One way to determine the numerical values of these intensities is to evaluate the sound wave by using a hydrophone. A hydrophone may be used by engineers to measure the output intensities as well as other characteristics of an ultrasound wave as well. The hydrophone is actually a transducer that is about the size of a needle that provides accurate values because of its compact size.

Types of Cavitation

The two types of cavitation that exist when the force and frequency from an ultrasound beam are applied to tissues are known as stable cavitation and transient cavitation. The mechanical index (MI) reading on the machine alerts the sonographer to the possibility that cavitation will create dangerous bioeffects within the tissue being imaged. A smaller MI number indicates that stable cavitation will occur. Stable cavitation is the increasing, decreasing, and vibration of gas bubbles located within tissue when it is exposed to variations in pressure of the sound wave. These bubbles tend to acquire much of the energy of the sound wave, but they do not rupture. Transient (normal,

Copyright © Mometrix Media. You have been licensed one copy of this document for personal use only. Any other reproduction or redistribution is strictly prohibited. All rights reserved.
This content is provided for test preparation purposes only and does not imply an endorsement by Mometrix of any particular political, scientific, or religious point of view.

inertial) cavitation occurs with higher MI readings. In this situation, the microbubbles tend to rupture, creating increased pressure and temperature measurements.

Beam Producing Greater Heating of Internal Tissue

A highly focused ultrasound beam can produce a greater degree of internal tissue heating because the energy of the beam is condensed into a thin region, especially at the focus where the beam diameter is already the smallest. Although this has a positive effect on image resolution, it may increase the internal temperature of tissue. Tissue heating relates to the spatial peak temporal average (SPTA) intensity. This is a value that should be watched closely by the operator, especially during fetal scans because bioeffects must be taken into consideration. When compared to an unfocused beam, a focused beam is allowed to have a higher SPTA limit because less tissue is being exposed. The intensity limit of a focused beam is set at 1 W/cm^2 or 1,000 mW/cm^2.

Applying the ALARA Principle to Decrease Patient Exposure

The as low as reasonably achievable (ALARA) principle is associated with radiation, but it is also an important rule for sonographers as well. For example, if an entire image is too bright, the most effective way to decrease patient exposure is to decrease the output power (also known as the acoustic power). By lowering the power, there is a decrease in the voltage applied to the ultrasound transducer, which, in turn, decreases the amount of energy that the patient is exposed to. A sonographer could also turn down the overall gain to prevent an image from being too bright but understand that gain has no effect on patient exposure. However, if an image is too dark, the best choice for adhering to the ALARA principle is to increase the gain because it does not affect the energy imparted to the patient.

Increasing Pixel Density to Improve an Image

A pixel refers to all of the tiny boxes that will each have their own gray shade in order to make up a digital image. In order to gain an image with greater resolution, a higher pixel density is required. Pixel density is the number of boxes per inch on the display. A high pixel density will offer better resolution because there will be more pixels found in every inch of the image. This, in turn, requires the pixels to be smaller which is what is desired when trying to improve the spatial resolution. If an image has a lower number of pixels, the pixels will be larger, so the spatial resolution will not be as great. This is considered to be a low-pixel-density image.

Parameters Increased When Operator Increases Output Power

Increasing the output power will have an impact on many parameters. One impact is that the sonographer will be afforded the opportunity to penetrate deeper in the body of the patient. Another parameter that is adjusted is the brightness of the image. When the output power is increased, the image becomes brighter throughout the entire display. If the output power is decreased, the overall image becomes darker. Increasing the output power will force the pulser component of the ultrasound machine to increase the amount of voltage that the PZT crystals receive in the transducers. This will create stronger pulses that are sent into the tissue, which in turn, creates an image that is brighter because of the amplified signals. It is important to note that output power is also referred to as acoustic power or output gain.

13-Microsecond Rule

Ultrasound machines are designed to calculate the speed of the ultrasound wave in soft tissue as 1.54 mm/μs. The time of flight refers to the time it takes for a pulse to leave the transducer, hit a reflector, and return back to the transducer. The depth of the reflector can be calculated as being 1 cm when the time of flight equals 13 μs. Using this rule, if a target is 2 cm deep, the time of flight will be twice as long, equating to 26 μs. If the time of flight is 39 μs, the depth of the reflector will be 3

Copyright © Mometrix Media. You have been licensed one copy of this document for personal use only. Any other reproduction or redistribution is strictly prohibited. All rights reserved.
This content is provided for test preparation purposes only and does not imply an endorsement by Mometrix of any particular political, scientific, or religious point of view.

cm. Sonographers should be aware of the reflector depth and the total distance traveled. For example, if a question states that the time of flight was 13 μs, and it is asked what the total distance traveled is, the answer would be 2 cm. At 13 μs, the depth would only be 1 cm, but the total distance would be $1\ cm + 1\ cm = 2\ cm$.

Time Gain Compensation Curve

A time gain compensation (TGC) curve has an x-axis as well as a y-axis. The horizontal x-axis refers to how much compensation is necessary for the depth of the object being imaged (y-axis). The top of the y-axis represents the patient's skin, and as it moves down, it refers to tissues that are located deeper in the body. The near gain is located superficially near the skin's surface. At this location, the structures being imaged need very little TGC because not much attenuation occurs. The slope is the middle portion of the TGC curve in which more compensation is necessary because of the greater depths. The knee is located at the distal portion of the slope and demonstrates where the most compensation will occur. The region of the far gain is distal to the knee at an ever-greater depth that also designates that the greatest amount of compensation has been offered by the machine.

Alternate Names for Overall Gain

Overall gain can also be referred to as receiver gain or the amplification of the ultrasound beam. It is a control on the ultrasound system that is used to produce a brighter or darker image. This control will affect the entire image. One should always keep the as low as reasonably achievable (ALARA) principle in mind because a sonographer can lessen the exposure to a patient if an image needs to be brightened by increasing the gain instead of the output power.

Units to Measure Compensation

Sonographers are aware of the term amplification. This refers to the brightness of an ultrasound signal. Amplification can be measured in decibels (dB). Compensation is a type of amplification, so it is also measured in dB. Amplification is the first process that takes place in the receiver. It will differentiate the strength of the beam as it enters and exits the receiver of the ultrasound system. The normal range for amplification of an image ranges from 60 to 100 dB. Changing only the amplification is not enough to create an image that is the same level of brightness throughout. The user must also consider adjusting the compensation. Compensation is the second process in the receiver and can be used in conjunction with amplification to create an image that demonstrates uniform brightness.

Reducing Shadowing and Speckle Artifacts

Spatial compounding is a technique that requires processing to average data that are obtained from multiple angles of interrogation. This method has proven to be successful in eliminating artifacts such as shadowing and speckle. Speckle artifacts are created when the ultrasound beam is scattered after interacting with various tissues. Noise that results from speckle artifacts will make the image appear grainy, but spatial compounding improves the signal-to-noise ratio, helping to eliminate some of the noise. Spatial compounding may also suppress the amount of shadowing that is apparent in an image. This is corrected because a single transducer is able to steer the frames from multiple directions and many angles will be perpendicular to the structures, decreasing the amount of shadowing.

Reject

Reject is the last process that takes place in the receiver. This function is typically offered in two forms: one that takes place automatically and one that can be controlled by the operator. The reject function enables the user to decide if low-level echoes should be displayed within the image. Sometimes, weaker signals will offer important data for a diagnosis, but clinicians do not want

Copyright © Mometrix Media. You have been licensed one copy of this document for personal use only. Any other reproduction or redistribution is strictly prohibited. All rights reserved.
This content is provided for test preparation purposes only and does not imply an endorsement by Mometrix of any particular political, scientific, or religious point of view.

noise to be present on the image. Stronger signals are not affected by reject. Some ultrasound manufactures will have other names for reject, such as suppression or threshold. Reject can decrease the amount of electronic noise that may be visualized while imaging the gallbladder or urinary bladder.

Effect of PRF on Imaging Depth and Range Ambiguity

Range ambiguity is an imaging error in which the echoes have not yet been returned to the transducer before the next pulse is transmitted. If the pulse repetition frequency (PRF) is too high while scanning a structure deep in the body, range ambiguity may occur. If this happens, the system will incorrectly place the received reflections closer to the probe than their actual depth. PRF represents the number of pulses sent into the body every second, and it is presented in units of hertz (Hz). The normal range of PRF or imaging systems is 1,000–10,000 Hz. If a sonographer increases the imaging depth, the system automatically decreases the PRF in order to avoid range ambiguity. In other words, the PRF is inversely related to the imaging depth; therefore, if the scan depth is twice as deep, the ultrasound system will automatically reduce the PRF by one-half.

Spatial Resolution and Pixel Density

Pixel stands for picture element. A pixel is the smallest portion of an image that is in a digital format. For example, a picture taken with a digital camera is made up of thousands of picture elements. Each pixel will consist of one color. Spatial resolution is a term that sonographers are familiar with, and this also applies to other digital technology. Pixel density refers to the number of pixels contained in every inch of the image. The more pixels that an image contains, the higher the spatial resolution will be. A high pixel density will dramatically improve an image whether it is on a digital camera, flat-screen TV, or ultrasound display. In this example, the terms "analog display" and "digital display" are added as additional information to throw the reader off, but if better spatial resolution is desired, the user must choose the 2000 × 2000 analog displays because of the higher pixel count.

Location of Analog-to-Digital Conversion

There are many components of an ultrasound system that are necessary to create an image. In order, the processes that take place are the pulser, beam former, receiver, memory, and image display screen. The pulser applies voltages to the transducer in order to excite the active elements within the probe. The functions of the pulser will take place during transmission of the ultrasound beam. The beam former controls the time delays when phased array technology is used. The receiver collects the returning signals from objects being imaged so that the data can, as an end result, be viewed on the image display screen. Memory is where the information is kept until it can be displayed on the ultrasound monitor. The analog-to-digital conversion has to take place between the transducer and the memory (also known as the scan converter). The analog signals received from the transducer must be digitized before they reach the memory of the system. A computer mouse is an example of an analog-to-digital conversion.

Location of Digital-to-Analog Conversion

There are many components of an ultrasound system that are necessary to create an image. In order, the processes that take place are the pulser, beam former, receiver, memory, and image display screen. The pulser applies voltages to the transducer in order to excite the active elements within the probe. The functions of the pulser will take place during transmission of the ultrasound beam. The beam former controls the time delays when phased-array technology is used. The receiver collects the returning signals from objects being imaged so that the data can, as an end result, be viewed on the image display screen. Memory is where the information is kept until it can be displayed on the ultrasound monitor. The digital-to-analog conversion has to take place between

Copyright © Mometrix Media. You have been licensed one copy of this document for personal use only. Any other reproduction or redistribution is strictly prohibited. All rights reserved.
This content is provided for test preparation purposes only and does not imply an endorsement by Mometrix of any particular political, scientific, or religious point of view.

the memory and the image display because the signal in the memory has to be changed into an analog signal to be displayed on the television monitor. An example of a digital-to-analog conversion is an iPod.

High Contrast

If the image displayed on an ultrasound system has a high amount of contrast, this means that the pixels are either black or white. In ultrasound images that are considered to be high contrast, very few shades of gray are visible. Sonographers should be familiar with the term dynamic range. This controls how the intensity of the signals is transformed into various shades of gray. This will either increase or limit the different shades of gray. In this example, if only black and white are created, then there is a narrow dynamic range. A dynamic range that shows many shades of gray would be considered a wide dynamic range. These images will be considered to be of low contrast. The dynamic range can be changed on the ultrasound system. If the user believes that the image is grainy, the dynamic range can be increased. If the image is too smooth, the user can increase the dynamic range.

Write Magnification

The type of magnification that is preferred because it offers improved spatial resolution is write magnification. Write magnification takes place before the data are stored in the scan converter. With this process of magnification, the area identified in the region of interest (ROI) is rescanned and the old data are ignored to obtain new information. This type of zoom increases the number of pixels when compared to the first image, which automatically increases the amount of spatial resolution. That is why this magnification process is the preferred method to zoom an image. Because it is completed before the data are stored in the scan converter, it cannot be performed after the image is frozen and is considered to be a preprocessing technique. Once rescanned, the temporal resolution may be improved if the new image is shallower than the original data.

Frequency Compounding

Frequency compounding is one method to reduce the amount of speckle in an ultrasound image. Ultrasound images, of course, are filled with speckle, but it is important that a reduction takes place in order to discern objects that demonstrate low contrast. Targets that are smaller may not be visualized if the amount of speckle is not reduced. Frequency compounding is an averaging method that tends to take the speckle patterns of multiple images into consideration to reduce the noise and speckle artifact that are present.

Edge Enhancement

If a sonographer wants to improve the sharpness of a mass located within the liver, edge enhancement can be applied. This is a technique that allows better delineation of the border of structures by sharpening the edges of a mass. Often, it is difficult to discern the differences in tissue types. Raising the image contrast at the interface of these tissues will enhance the change that may not be as obvious without edge enhancement. At the boundary between two or more tissue types, various shades of gray are displayed, and edge enhancement will produce edges that are more reflective to help the mass stand out against normal liver tissue. Edge enhancement can also be helpful when imaging uterine fibroids or masses within the thyroid.

Read Magnification

Magnification allows users to zoom in or increase the size of a region of interest. Read magnification is performed after an image has already been stored in the scan converter; it allows for postprocessing function because it can enlarge an image that has been frozen, but the spatial resolution tends to stay the same because the magnified image still contains the same number of

Copyright © Mometrix Media. You have been licensed one copy of this document for personal use only. Any other reproduction or redistribution is strictly prohibited. All rights reserved.
This content is provided for test preparation purposes only and does not imply an endorsement by Mometrix of any particular political, scientific, or religious point of view.

pixels as the original image. The image is not reconstructed by the system; the pixels are just larger than they were in the first image. This function has no effect on the frame rate (temporal resolution) because the image will be located at the same depth as the original information. Because the spatial resolution is not any better than the original image, this is not the preferred method of magnification.

3D Rendering

Postprocessing allows ultrasound users to manage information after it has been stored in the ultrasound system's scan converter. For example, anything that a sonographer does to a frozen image is a postprocessing technique. All postprocessing applications can be undone because the original data are saved. The 3D rendering is one example of a postprocessing technique. The data are required, and the image is either reconstructed on the ultrasound system or it is sent to an offline workstation that is equipped with special software to manipulate and analyze the images. Other examples of postprocessing would be to adjust the gain after an image is frozen or to magnify the image after it has been frozen.

Fusion Imaging

Fusion imaging (also known as hybrid imaging) is a technique that provides sonographers and clinicians with greater diagnostic confidence when following up lesions discovered on previous computed tomography (CT) or magnetic resonance imaging (MRI) studies. Fusion imaging also reduces the amount of radiation that a patient is exposed to because ultrasound does not use radiation. Still another advantage is greater dynamic monitoring during invasive procedures. Real-time virtual sonography is one example of hybrid imaging that allows gray-scale, color Doppler, or the use of contrast harmonics and CT or MRI images to be displayed simultaneously. The CT or MRI images must be sent to the ultrasound system so that the same cross-sectional image can be recreated with sonography. Fusion imaging requires a sensor that is attached to the transducer that determines the probe location during the scan as well as a transmitter that is attached to the patient.so the sonographer knows the suspicious lesion is being evaluated.

Visualizing the Abdominal Aorta

If the radiologist would like to visualize as much of the abdominal aorta as possible, the sonographer could use the extended field of view control on the ultrasound system. This panoramic image is available on most modern ultrasound equipment and replaces the split-screen method of demonstrating objects that are longer than the transducer face. By acquiring various volume data, the system will stitch the information together in order to display one image. This single image will offer clinicians the ability to visualize the structure at the same time. This application can be used when interrogating the abdominal aorta, and it may provide additional information regarding the exact location of aneurysms that may be encountered. Often, anatomical structures are enlarged, and it may be difficult to obtain measurements from them. These include the thyroid, testes, polycystic kidneys, musculoskeletal exams, as well as some breast lesions.

3D Ultrasound Technology

Three- and four-dimensional (3D and 4D) ultrasound exams are performed with a 2D array transducer. This is also referred to as volume imaging because once a good 2D image is created, the transducer will allow volume data acquisition when turning on 3D or 4D. These transducers are able to obtain volume data with the complex arrangement of the active elements. Thousands of active elements are arranged across the transducer face. They are not only situated vertically, but also in a horizontal line across the transducer. The 2D array probes allow for the sound beams to be electronically steered and focused beams. This design in the arrangement of the crystals will result in extremely thin slices of the sound beam when compared to traditional transducers. The thin

Copyright © Mometrix Media. You have been licensed one copy of this document for personal use only. Any other reproduction or redistribution is strictly prohibited. All rights reserved.
This content is provided for test preparation purposes only and does not imply an endorsement by Mometrix of any particular political, scientific, or religious point of view.

slices enable better contrast resolution because the beam is not wider than the structure being interrogated. Contrast resolution is augmented due to diminished volume averaging.

Two-Dimensional Transducers

Two-dimensional transducers (2D arrays) offer a fairly recent technology that is continuing to be developed and improved. These 2D transducers are used to create 3D and 4D images. These probes contain thousands of piezoelectric elements arranged in what can be compared to the shape of a checkerboard. These beams are electronically focused and steered in order to obtain volume data. A 3D rendering can then be performed on the data collected to create the 3D images. This 3D technique is considered to be postprocessing because the computer-generated images are manipulated. This technology is used in obstetrical ultrasound as well as diagnostic imaging for various diseases and disorders on nonpregnant populations. For example, 3D and 4D have proved useful during pelvic ultrasounds looking at the uterus and the ovaries. They can also be applied to abdominal exams to better discern liver, renal, or adrenal masses.

Grayscale Imaging

The most basic form of real-time or grayscale imaging is known as brightness mode. This method is more commonly referred to as B-mode imaging. B-mode was the first gray-scale imaging method available. During B-mode, pulses are sent into the body and when the signal returns, it appears as a dot on the screen. The amplitude or strength of the reflectors will be visualized as dots. Higher amplitudes will appear as bright-white areas on the screen. The areas that return weaker signals will be seen as gray dots on the image display. Even when color mode is used, the underlying image showing the actual anatomy of the patient is represented by grayscale imaging.

Echotextures

Various organs, tissues, glands, cysts, and masses can be interrogated with ultrasound technology, and they will display a typical echotexture. Radiologists will comment on the size and echotextures of these structures in their reports to give the ordering physician additional information to help reach a diagnosis. Common ultrasound terms associated with echotexture include cystic, solid, complex, homogeneous, and heterogeneous. Ultrasound is often used when a mass is felt or suspected to determine if it is cystic (fluid-filled), solid (not cystic), or complex (containing cystic and solid components). Other common terms used when describing organs and glands are homogeneous (uniform echo pattern) and heterogeneous (uneven echo patterns). Some diseases, such as cirrhosis of the liver, will change the normal echotexture of the liver and be referred to as a coarse echotexture. In this case, the typical smooth appearance is no longer evident.

Variance Mode Map

A variance mode map gives the sonographer information not only about the direction and velocity of red blood cells in the sample, but also about the flow pattern of the blood. Similar to velocity mode maps, variance mode maps have a black line that represents where no Doppler shift occurs. Above this black line is flow moving toward the probe, and below the black line is flow moving away from the probe. However, the boxes above and below the black line contain different colors on each side. Recall that normal flow in a vessel is considered laminar flow, which is represented by flow on the left of the color map. Turbulent flow is the opposite of laminar flow and is found on the right side of the color map. An example of turbulent flow may be the result of blood flow moving through a stenotic vessel.

Aliasing Artifact

Aliasing is an imaging error that occurs when a sonographer is interrogating a structure with Doppler ultrasound. Although power Doppler imaging (PDI) is a special form of color Doppler, it

Copyright © Mometrix Media. You have been licensed one copy of this document for personal use only. Any other reproduction or redistribution is strictly prohibited. All rights reserved.
This content is provided for test preparation purposes only and does not imply an endorsement by Mometrix of any particular political, scientific, or religious point of view.

only indicates that a Doppler shift has taken place. It does not examine the velocity (speed and direction) of the moving blood cells, but rather the strength of the signal (amplitude). Because there are not any data pertaining to the velocity, aliasing will not occur. This is just one advantage of the use of PDI. PDI is more sensitive than color Doppler, so it is often used to visualize blood flow within smaller vessels or areas of venous (low) flow.

Blood Flow During an Echocardiogram

An echocardiogram is an ultrasound exam that evaluates various structures of the heart. The movement of blood flow as it travels through the heart is also observed, and measurements can be taken. Hemodynamics refers to the observation of blood flow as it courses through the heart and blood vessels. During an echocardiogram, the ultrasound user would expect to visualize blood flow that is pulsatile. The heart is constantly contracting and relaxing, which will create velocities of blood flow that will fluctuate because of the movement of the heart wall. Pulsatile flow is also visualized in the arterial system because blood is moving at a greater velocity than it is in the venous system.

Adjusting PRF to Maximize Visualization of Rapid Blood Flow and Reduce Aliasing

Correct optimization of color flow is always the goal when examining vessels while using color Doppler. In order to get the entire vessel to fill in properly, one of the first steps that the sonographer can perform after turning on the color flow is to adjust the pulse repetition frequency (PRF). The PRF is often referred to as the color scale when color Doppler is activated. In this example, the blood flow is moving at a rapid pace, and it is likely in an artery, so the ultrasound user would want to increase the PRF. This raises the Nyquist limit of the machine, which will help avoid aliasing. Aliasing can occur in color Doppler imaging and will appear as a variety of colors within the lumen of the blood vessel. The next step the sonographer may take is to increase the color gain if the vessel is not completely filled with color.

Continuous-Wave (CW) Transducer Sensitivity

Dedicated continuous-wave (CW) transducers cannot produce an ultrasound image, but they have a heightened sensitivity to blood flow. The reason that they are more prone to signals that are weaker within the body is because these probes do not contain backing (damping) material. Backing material inhibits the amount of ringing of the crystals during the transmitting and receiving phases, which makes them less receptive to receiving returning signals that tend to be smaller. If these tiny signals are not recognized by the transducer, then the ultrasound system cannot convert them into electrical signals to be visualized on the screen. Dedicated continuous-wave probes are great tools to detect tiny Doppler shifts such as blood flow in the foot. Matching layers are, however, present in dedicated continuous-wave probes to allow for the propagation of sound in and out of the body more readily.

Optimal Setting for Color Doppler Gain

If a sonographer visualizes multiple speckled colors throughout the color box after turning on color Doppler, the first step that he or she can take to correct this noise is to turn the color gain down. Color gain that is set correctly is adjusted so that the amplitude is set at the highest level without displaying color speckles. Aliasing, color Doppler gain that is set too high, and turbulent flow all have different appearances, so ultrasound users should be able to discern what is taking place. Some are artifacts and can be corrected with the adjustment of parameters on the ultrasound machine.

Copyright © Mometrix Media. You have been licensed one copy of this document for personal use only. Any other reproduction or redistribution is strictly prohibited. All rights reserved.
This content is provided for test preparation purposes only and does not imply an endorsement by Mometrix of any particular political, scientific, or religious point of view.

Laminar Flow

Laminar flow is the type of flow that is exhibited in normal anatomical structures. If a clinician listens to the blood moving through a vessel with laminar flow, it will not be heard. This flow is layered, smooth, and travels parallel along the length of the vessel. There are two configurations regarding laminar flow. The first is plug flow, which will have the same velocity in all layers present. A parabolic pattern tends to have velocities that are higher in the middle of the vessel and lower velocity flow along the walls. The shape that is created with a parabolic flow pattern is similar to a bullet. A blood vessel that contains laminar flow will produce a Reynolds number of less than 1,500. The Reynolds number is a way to forecast if the flow will be laminar or turbulent. Turbulent flow will have a Reynolds number that is greater than 2,000.

Advantages and Disadvantages of a Larger Packet Size

Packet size should be carefully evaluated so that color Doppler velocities can be interrogated more accurately. The advantages of a larger packet size include a heightened receptiveness to blood vessels that have blood flow that is moving at a slower velocity. Another advantage is that when the packet size is larger, more pulses are sent out for every scan line that is available, and in turn the velocity measurements of the blood flow tend to be more precise. The disadvantages are that because more pulses are required for larger packet sizes, the frame rate and temporal resolution will be degraded because more processing time is required by the system.

Disadvantages of Persistence

Persistence (also called temporal averaging or temporal compounding) is a method that can be used during grayscale or color Doppler imaging. By overlapping information obtained from older frames onto more recent images obtained, the machine can produce an ultrasound image with greater detail that has less noise, is smoother, and has a higher signal-to-noise ratio. If the signal-to-noise ratio is higher than the noise, the system will get rid of the noise signals. Although the image detail improves with the use of temporal compounding, the temporal resolution is degraded because of the additional processing. This makes imaging structures that are moving rapidly very difficult because there will be a lag as the temporal resolution is decreased. Persistence is best used with structures that demonstrate slow motion.

Transducers Offering Pulsed-Wave Doppler

Pulsed-wave Doppler only requires one active element. This lead zirconate titanate (PZT) crystal is able to transmit the pulse into the body as well as listen for the returning signals. Only one PZT crystal is necessary because the sonographer places the sample volume (gate) in exactly the position at which a sample velocity is necessary. Once the probe transmits a pulse into the body, it listens for it to return to the transducer. This is known as the time of flight (go-return time). Transducers that allow pulsed Doppler are also able to create a grayscale image. This is referred to as duplex/triplex imaging. A duplex/triplex exam consists of gray scale, color Doppler, and pulsed-wave Doppler. In contrast, a continuous-wave transducer will consist of two crystals. One active element serves as a transmitter that introduces pulses into the body at a constant rate. The second active element acts as a receiver for the returning echoes.

Advantage of Range Resolution

Range resolution allows ultrasound users to select the exact region where a pulsed-wave Doppler sample should take place. Range resolution is also called range specificity because a specific location is chosen. Perhaps this area is where a stenosis is visualized on grayscale images, so the sonographer must obtain a measurement within the stenotic portion of the vessel as well as check for turbulence distal to this location. When pulsed-wave Doppler is activated, the gate (sample

Copyright © Mometrix Media. You have been licensed one copy of this document for personal use only. Any other reproduction or redistribution is strictly prohibited. All rights reserved.
This content is provided for test preparation purposes only and does not imply an endorsement by Mometrix of any particular political, scientific, or religious point of view.

volume) will appear on the screen and it can be quickly moved to the location of interest. Continuous-wave Doppler does not offer range resolution because the sample is being obtained from every vessel that is in the path of the ultrasound wave. This is superior to pulsed-wave Doppler when measuring vessels that have an extremely high velocity, but range ambiguity occurs with continuous-wave Doppler.

Range Ambiguity

Recall that range ambiguity artifact (also known as range specificity or range resolution) is typically prevented when an ultrasound operator uses pulsed-wave Doppler. During these exams, a sample volume is used to determine the exact location in which a velocity measurement should be obtained. However, in this example, if the pulse repetition frequency (PRF) (scale) is set too high for the depth of the reflector being interrogated, range ambiguity will exist because the system will be directed to send out pulses before the earlier pulses have been returned. If the echoes are not returned in the order that they are transmitted, the system will incorrectly determine the depth of the object being scanned because this is assumed by the ultrasound system. In this case, aliasing will occur, which can be corrected by increasing the scale.

Importance of PRF and the Nyquist Limit

Sonographers should recognize the Nyquist limit as the greatest velocity of blood flow that can be measured just before aliasing occurs. Aliasing is when the color or spectral Doppler patterns wind around the display. The pulse repetition frequency (PRF) can be referred to as the velocity scale, and it plays an important role in eliminating aliasing. When the sonographer modifies the PRF, the Nyquist limit automatically changes as well. There is a direct relationship between the PRF and the Nyquist limit. When the PRF scale is as high as it can go, the likelihood of aliasing occurring is slim. A scale that is set low will have a lower Nyquist limit with a greater chance of aliasing.

Advantage of Continuous-Wave Doppler

The main advantage of using continuous-wave Doppler on an ultrasound system is that precise velocity measurements can be obtained because two crystals are used instead of one. The crystals are constantly and simultaneously transmitting an ultrasound pulse while one is always listening or receiving a signal. When using a nonimaging continuous-wave probe, the sensitivity is increased because this probe can detect very small Doppler frequencies because it doesn't contain a dampening (backing) layer. Both of these types of continuous-wave devices have a matching layer to make them more proficient in sending and receiving pulses. Continuous-wave Doppler will never display aliasing because only pulsed-wave Doppler will alias. One major disadvantage is that there isn't a sample gate, so the precise location of where the velocities are located is not known.

Measuring Blood Flow Velocity

The method used to measure the velocity of blood flow within the body is called the Doppler principle. The frequency of sound varies as the distance between the transmitted frequency and receiver change positions. If the distance between the sound source and receiver stays the same, the frequency will not be altered. An alteration of the frequency is called a Doppler shift or Doppler frequency. The Doppler shift is directly related to the velocity of blood within the circulatory system. Keep in mind that the velocity includes the speed (magnitude) and direction of blood flow. Slower velocities will cause a lower Doppler frequency. A higher velocity will create a greater Doppler shift. Blood flow velocities are reported in units of meters per second (m/s).

Copyright © Mometrix Media. You have been licensed one copy of this document for personal use only. Any other reproduction or redistribution is strictly prohibited. All rights reserved.
This content is provided for test preparation purposes only and does not imply an endorsement by Mometrix of any particular political, scientific, or religious point of view.

Reynolds Number

The Reynolds number is a value that predicts the onset of flow that is turbulent. The Reynolds number is a unitless value that is calculated from the following equation:

$$Reynolds\ number = \frac{average\ flow\ speed \times vessel\ diameter \times density}{viscosity}$$

If the calculated value is less than 1,500, laminar flow will be present. If the value is more than 2,000, it is predicted that a turbulent flow will be visualized. Disturbed flow will fall between the 1,500 and 2,000 range. From the above equation, if there is an increased speed of flow, there will be a higher Reynolds number. If the diameter of the vessel is larger, the Reynolds number will also be greater. Density has the same effect on the Reynolds number. The Reynolds number has an indirect relationship with the viscosity of the blood.

Phasic vs. Steady Flow

Three types of blood flow that are witnessed in the circulatory systems of humans are phasic, pulsatile, and steady flow. Phasic flow is the typical flow pattern seen in veins. Phasic flow will exhibit velocity changes associated with breathing that causes red blood cells to speed up or slow down. Steady flow is constantly present in the venous system, and it takes place when the patient holds their breath. Steady flow does not vary in velocity, but rather it moves at the same speed. No acceleration or deceleration is present due to the contraction of the heart.

Doppler Shift Range

When using ultrasound for diagnostic purposes, the frequency of the transducers used during a Doppler exam ranges from approximately 2 to 10 MHz. This question asks about the range in which a Doppler shift takes place. This falls in the audible range in which sound can actually be heard, which is anywhere between 20 Hz and 20,000 Hz. The formula to calculate a Doppler shift is as follows:

$$Doppler\ shift\ =\ reflected\ frequency - transmtted\ frequency.$$

Remember that Doppler shift is often referred to as Doppler frequency, and it provides information pertaining to velocity.

Using Color Flow Imaging

Blood is composed of many components including red blood cells (erythrocytes), white blood cells (leukocytes), platelets (thrombocytes), and plasma. Roughly 45 percent of the blood that travels throughout the circulatory system (heart, arteries, capillaries, and veins) is comprised of red blood cells. Red blood cells supply oxygen to all of the cells in the body and are the most numerous type of cell in whole blood. The life span of red blood cells is about 120 days, but they are constantly being replenished with new red blood cells. Because red blood cells are traveling in the heart and blood vessels, they create the reflections that are seen by the human eye when color Doppler is turned on (sometimes the blood flow can be seen, especially in low-flow states without color Doppler). Color Doppler should also be used when scanning a mass to demonstrate if the flow pattern is within or around the perimeter of the lesion.

Angle(s) Providing the Greatest Amount of Doppler Shift

If a sonographer is using pulsed-wave Doppler in order to determine the peak velocity of blood flow in a vessel, the operator must remember that when the red blood cells are moving along the same path of the ultrasound beam, the most accurate measurements will be obtained. Thus, the Doppler

Copyright © Mometrix Media. You have been licensed one copy of this document for personal use only. Any other reproduction or redistribution is strictly prohibited. All rights reserved.
This content is provided for test preparation purposes only and does not imply an endorsement by Mometrix of any particular political, scientific, or religious point of view.

shift (otherwise known as the Doppler frequency) will be highest at 0 or 180 degrees. This parallel movement can be either toward or away from the transducer, but in this case the entire velocity of the moving particles will be measured with 100% certainty. If the angle between the target and reflector is anything other than 0 or 180 degrees, the velocity is less precise. If an operator tries to interrogate a structure at a 90-degree angle with pulsed-wave Doppler, no Doppler shift will take place because it is calculated to be zero.

Differentiating Between Flow Reversal and Aliasing with Color Doppler

It is important for sonographers to realize that aliasing can occur not only with spectral Doppler analysis, but also with color flow Doppler. The user must be able to discern between aliasing and the reversal of flow (bidirectional flow). In order to determine if aliasing is present, the user must pay close attention to the color map located on the side of the image. If the colors on the map tend to wrap from the top around the outside and to the bottom of the map, then users may assume that aliasing is present. If the colors on the middle of the color map communicate with each other, then bidirectional flow is present. The best step that an ultrasound user can take in order to remove an aliasing artifacts from a color Doppler exam is to increase the level of the velocity scale.

Pulsed-Wave Doppler

When performing a pulsed-wave Doppler exam, the user is able to determine exactly where a velocity measurement should be taken within a vessel. Once the sonographer has the grayscale image optimized, color Doppler can be activated to better visualize the blood vessels. Then, one can bring up the cursor for pulsed-wave Doppler and a line that is intersected by two dashes close together will be visualized. This is the gate (sample volume). The gate can be moved with the trackball until it is right where the user wants to perform a spectral analysis. The size of the gate can be changed so that it is only within the vessel that is being examined. For example, if one is sampling the carotid artery but the spectral display is also showing venous flow, reduce the size of the gate and reposition it so that only the artery is being interrogated.

Spectral Broadening

A spectral Doppler waveform represents all of the many velocities found in a sample of a blood vessel. Two types of flow can be ascertained in the sample. They are normal or laminar flow, in which the spectral window is clear and the red blood cells are traveling at almost the same velocities. Turbulent flow shows flow that is disorganized because the blood is traveling at different speeds and various directions. Instead of a clear spectral window as seen in laminar flow, it appears to be filled in, which represents spectral broadening. Spectral broadening is a display of a broad range of Doppler shifts that are apparent within the sample of blood flow taken in a vessel. This may happen due to a stenosis or tortuous vessel.

Spectral Doppler Gain

Pulsed-wave Doppler provides important information that can be used to diagnose many disorders in patients. Correct Doppler settings are crucial, and sonographers must have a strong understanding of not only anatomy, but also ultrasound physics. If the machine is not set properly, an artifact can occur that may limit the amount of diagnostic information present. If a sonographer turns on the pulsed-wave Doppler, but the spectral display can barely be visualized, then the next step will be to turn up the pulsed-wave Doppler's gain. If the gain is turned up too high, then noise may appear in the spectral display. One can increase the gain by turning it up until noise appears. At this point, the gain may be slowly reduced until the noise disappears.

Copyright © Mometrix Media. You have been licensed one copy of this document for personal use only. Any other reproduction or redistribution is strictly prohibited. All rights reserved.
This content is provided for test preparation purposes only and does not imply an endorsement by Mometrix of any particular political, scientific, or religious point of view.

Resistance Index

Recall that arteries are the blood vessels that supply organs with oxygenated blood. These arteries are able to direct the flow of blood to the organs that require more blood such as the brain, liver, kidneys, and gonads. These arteries can control the resistance of the blood flow so that it is routed to those organs. The term RI refers to the resistance (or resistivity) index, and it is a number that can be calculated by today's ultrasound machines to measure this resistance to blood flow. Low-resistance flow is seen in arteries that supply organs that need a constant source of blood flow such as the internal carotid, hepatic, and renal arteries. High arterial resistance demonstrates arterioles that have constricted and created a channeling to reroute the blood flow elsewhere. Examples of high-resistance vessels include the external carotid arteries, mesenteric arteries in a patient that is fasting, and arteries that supply the limbs. Sonographers should be aware that the normal value for RI will be different from one artery to the next, but anything above or below the typical values may be an abnormal finding.

Spectral Analysis

Spectral analysis is the method that provides information pertaining to the individual velocities of blood cells that are contained within a specific sample. Spectral analysis is a tool that simplifies the many Doppler shifts that are produced when blood travels through the body. Blood does not travel in a uniform fashion, and because of this, spectral analysis is necessary to provide data that can offer diagnostic information in order to correctly diagnosis patients that suffer from vascular disease. Sonographers realize that even within the same blood vessel that is free of any pathology, the blood moves at different speeds. When pathology is present, or the vessels change shapes and sizes, the flow patterns can change dramatically. Spectral analysis is a great tool that allows users to visually sort out all of this information along with measuring various velocities.

Nyquist Limit with Pulsed-Wave Doppler

The Nyquist limit can be calculated by dividing the pulse repetition frequency (PRF) by 2. Aliasing will be apparent if the Doppler frequency is higher than the Nyquist limit. Therefore, in order to prevent aliasing, the sonographer should raise the Nyquist limit. This can be done by raising the PRF (also known as the scale); if the PRF is increased, so is the Nyquist limit. One may also raise the Nyquist limit by finding a new sonographic window that is at a shallower location. The PRF is determined by the depth of the reflector. If the depth is deeper in the body, the PRF will be low, as will the Nyquist limit. This decreased value makes the ultrasound system more susceptible to aliasing.

Wall Filter

The wall filter is an important tool that sonographers can use in order to remove Doppler shifts below a certain set frequency during spectral and color Doppler interrogations. In other words, this control will help remove the lower frequency Doppler signals that may arise from the motion that anatomical structures such as the heart or blood vessels create. Wall filters are also referred to as high-pass filters and do not play a role in higher Doppler shifts such as those created from the movement of blood cells in the circulatory system. Sonographers should remember that blood that is moving slower will create a lower frequency Doppler shift. The system is less likely to detect blood that is moving slowly when the wall filter is set at a higher level.

Velocities That Are below the Baseline

When using spectral analysis to determine the velocity of blood flow and flow velocities are below the baseline, this represents blood cells that are traveling in a direction away from the transducer. Aliasing is an error in imaging that can represent high-velocity flows to wrap around the baseline

Copyright © Mometrix Media. You have been licensed one copy of this document for personal use only. Any other reproduction or redistribution is strictly prohibited. All rights reserved.
This content is provided for test preparation purposes only and does not imply an endorsement by Mometrix of any particular political, scientific, or religious point of view.

and appear as if they are moving in the opposite direction. An advantage of pulsed Doppler is that the user knows exactly where the blood flow velocity is being sampled because of the gate. Color flow Doppler allows information pertaining to the velocities to be superimposed on a grayscale image. Color flow Doppler also allows users to determine in which direction the blood is traveling.

Ring-down Artifact

A ring-down artifact is indicative of abdominal gas pockets such as those seen in pneumobilia (the presence of gas in the biliary ducts). It appears as a solid streak (or parallel bands) radiating away from the gas pocket itself.

Comet-Tail Artifact

The comet-tail artifact appears as multiple, small, white streaks running parallel to the target structure. It is caused by the reflection of the ultrasound beam off of small, spherical, reflective objects (such as gas bubbles or stones).

Refraction Artifacts

Refraction is ultrasound beam bending that occurs when the incident beam is not perpendicular to the target structure. It commonly occurs where bone meets soft tissue. Refraction may produce images that are not viewed in their correct positions on the ultrasound monitor. This may result in an inability to accurately measure characteristics such as length or depth.

Reverberation Artifacts

Reverberation occurs when the ultrasound beam reflects off of tissues that have different levels of acoustic impedance (resistance to vibration). Reverberations appear as equally spaced, bright rings that decrease in brightness as the transducer face moves away.

Mirror Artifact

A mirror artifact will always be visualized at a depth greater than that of the actual structure being imaged. It is known as a mirror artifact because a very strong reflector tends to redirect the sound waves as it strikes the mirror. This mirror will appear between the actual object being imaged and the second copy of the structure. The second copy will be equidistant from the reflector as the object, but it will be at a greater depth. This artifact can appear not only in grayscale imaging, but also during color Doppler interrogation. In this case, a second vessel may appear deeper than the actual vessel, but it is actually a mirror artifact. When imaging the abdomen, a common mirror imaging artifact visualized is lung tissue on either side of the diaphragm, which is seen as a bright reflector.

Edge Shadow Artifact

A shadow protruding from the edge of a curved structure that is parallel to the axis of the ultrasound beam is referred to as an edge shadow. These are hypoechoic or anechoic structures that may prevent the sonographer from visualizing underlying anatomical structures. These artifacts are created from a decrease in intensity as a sound beam refracts and diverges at the same time after making contact with a curved reflector. These artifacts are often seen when performing an ultrasound of a cyst or during a testicular scan.

Appearance of Enhancement and Shadowing Artifacts

Clinicians may use ultrasound artifacts as a tool to increase diagnostic confidence. For example, if a structure is fluid filled, posterior enhancement should be visualized posterior to the cyst. Anything that is filled with fluid will appear anechoic because it has a lower attenuation rate. The surrounding tissue that is below anything that is fluid filled will appear brighter and is known as an

Copyright © Mometrix Media. You have been licensed one copy of this document for personal use only. Any other reproduction or redistribution is strictly prohibited. All rights reserved.
This content is provided for test preparation purposes only and does not imply an endorsement by Mometrix of any particular political, scientific, or religious point of view.

enhancement artifact. While evaluating the ovaries, the enhancement artifact helps clinicians discern that the structure is fluid filled. Shadowing is the opposite of an enhancement artifact; this is a hypoechoic area posterior to a highly attenuating structure. This hypoechoic area prevents users from being able to see any underlying anatomy to these objects, but it provides clues of stones or calcifications. Sonographers may visualize small calcifications within the ovary, artery, or even within blood vessels.

Refraction Artifact

Refraction is the bending of a sound beam when it travels from one medium to another. Two conditions must occur in order for refraction to take place in a clinical setting: (1) There must be an oblique incidence, and (2) the two media must be traveling at different speeds because refraction cannot take place if they have identical speeds. Clinically, an ultrasound beam will only bend slightly at various tissue interfaces. Bone tends to create larger refraction angles because the speed of ultrasound in bone is faster than the speed of sound in soft tissues. Snell's law is used to calculate refraction, and the following equation may be used:

$$\frac{\sin(angle\ of\ transmission)}{\sin(angle\ of\ incidence)} = \frac{speed\ of\ medium\ 2}{speed\ of\ medium\ 1}$$

Visualizing Edge Shadowing

When a sonographer visualizes a shadow protruding from the edge of a curved structure that is parallel to the axis of the ultrasound beam, it may be referred to as an edge shadow. These artifacts are portrayed as thin, hypoechoic structures that may actually prevent a user from visualizing underlying anatomical structures. These artifacts are created from a decrease in intensity as a sound beam refracts and diverges at the same time after making contact with a curved reflector. Refraction will take place when the propagation speeds are different in the presence of oblique incidence. These artifacts are often seen when performing an ultrasound of a cyst or during a testicular scan. Other examples may include a transverse image of the gallbladder or fetal head due to the curvature of these structures.

Enhancement Artifact

While imaging a structure that is fluid filled, for example, a cyst or the gallbladder, the tissue that is visualized posterior to these structures often appears extremely echogenic. The artifact that is the opposite of shadowing is known as an enhancement artifact. These fluid-filled structures visualized are the result of a lower rate of attenuation than the tissue that surrounds them, so structures below them may appear brighter. Shadowing produces a hypoechoic area behind an object that is highly attenuating, and it can prohibit visualization of the structures that extend underneath these structures. Enhancement can be of diagnostic value because radiologists rely on this enhancement artifact to reassure them that a structure is cystic.

Shadowing Artifact

Shadowing is visualized when a highly attenuating structure is situated just above this artifact. Shadowing artifacts can often prevent the user from seeing underlying anatomical structures, but they may also serve as a helpful diagnostic indicator during ultrasound exams. A shadowing artifact appears as a hypoechoic or anechoic area deep to the structure that is highly attenuating. Sonographers may notice shadowing posterior to calcifications such as kidney stones and gallstones to aid the radiologist in making a correct diagnosis. The artifact that appears completely different than those characteristics of a shadowing artifact is known as enhancement. Enhancement also provides diagnostic value because radiologists rely on this enhancement artifact to reassure them that a structure is cystic. In this case, a hyperechoic region appears deep to a structure that is

Copyright © Mometrix Media. You have been licensed one copy of this document for personal use only. Any other reproduction or redistribution is strictly prohibited. All rights reserved.
This content is provided for test preparation purposes only and does not imply an endorsement by Mometrix of any particular political, scientific, or religious point of view.

weakly attenuating. For example, while imaging a cyst or the gallbladder, the tissue that is visualized posterior to these structures often appears extremely echogenic. Artifacts often seen during a testicular scan or while imaging cysts are edge shadows. They are the result of a decrease in intensity as a sound beam refracts and diverges at the same time after making contact with a curved reflector.

Flash Artifact

A disadvantage of power Doppler imaging (PDI) is that the study may suffer because of flash artifact. Flash artifact occurs not because of the motion of the red blood cells, but rather it is a burst of color visualized when there is motion taking place outside of the blood vessels. Often, this motion is caused by patient motion. Examples of patient motion may be that the patient is actually moving on the exam table, but it may also be involuntary motion such as movement of the heart or lungs during respiration. Flash artifact may also appear because of motion caused by the transducer as the sonographer is moving it on the patient or even motion caused from the pressure that the transducer places on soft-tissue structures. Flash artifact may appear as a randomized burst of color, occurring outside of the vessels.

Intermittent Sampling and Aliasing Artifacts

Aliasing is common during pulsed-wave Doppler exams due to intermittent sampling. Intermittent sampling occurs if the Doppler frequency is not evaluated correctly. When the Doppler frequency is larger than the Nyquist limit, which is equal to half of the pulse repetition frequency (PRF), then aliasing will take place. Aliasing is when the blood flow direction is incorrectly portrayed either above or below the baseline; it will wind around the entire spectral window and appear to move in the opposite direction. Aliasing can also arise when color flow Doppler is being used, so ultrasound users should be able to identify if it is present. Aliasing will never occur with continuous-wave Doppler because it can only be the result of pulsed ultrasound technology.

Aliasing with Color Doppler

Color Doppler uses grayscale imaging to locate the anatomical structures, and when activated, a color box will be layered on top of the B-mode image. This information includes data about the mean velocity of blood moving through various structures instead of peak velocity as measured by pulsed-wave and continuous-wave Doppler. Color Doppler does provide information regarding the direction of blood flow, and it is prone to aliasing. Ultrasound users should be able to tell the difference between color Doppler that is aliasing and flow that is moving in the reverse direction. The operator must pay close attention to the color map displayed on the screen. Just as pulsed-wave Doppler that is aliasing tends to wrap around the spectral window, color Doppler that is aliasing winds around the top of the color box around to the bottom.

Correcting an Aliasing Artifact During a Carotid Duplex Exam

Spectral Doppler waveforms can provide clinicians with a lot of insight pertaining to blood flowing throughout the body. Blood does not necessarily travel in the same speed or direction, even within the same blood vessel. Spectral analysis is a tool that identifies every velocity obtained within the signal that is reflected. However, when there are aliasing errors in the spectral waveform, the interpreting physician may mistake that data as true information. This could lead to a misdiagnosis. In this example, a 10 MHz transducer is creating an aliasing artifact so the sonographer may try to reduce the transducer's Doppler frequency. The PRF scale could also be increased to raise the Nyquist limit, and the baseline could be moved down. If that doesn't work, the user could increase the angle of incidence or switch to continuous-wave Doppler.

Copyright © Mometrix Media. You have been licensed one copy of this document for personal use only. Any other reproduction or redistribution is strictly prohibited. All rights reserved.
This content is provided for test preparation purposes only and does not imply an endorsement by Mometrix of any particular political, scientific, or religious point of view.

Doppler Gain Artifacts

Doppler gain artifacts must be corrected so that data are not lost or misinterpreted. In order to get the entire vessel to fill in properly, one of the first steps that the sonographer can perform after turning on color flow is to adjust the pulse repetition frequency (PRF), which is often referred to as the color scale when color Doppler is activated. In arteries, the blood is flowing rapidly, so the ultrasound user would want to increase the PRF. This raises the Nyquist limit of the machine, which will help avoid aliasing. Aliasing can occur in color Doppler imaging and will appear as a variety of colors within the lumen of the blood vessel. The next step the sonographer may take is to increase the color gain if the vessel is not completely filled with color. Color Doppler is often used during venous duplex exams of the extremities. In this example, the sonographer is trying to optimize color flow in the smaller vessels of a patient's lower leg. If color flow is not immediately visualized after turning on color Doppler, the sonographer should adjust the PRF, otherwise known as the color scale.

Aliasing Artifact

Spectral analysis is a tool that identifies every velocity obtained within the signal that is reflected. However, when there are aliasing errors in the spectral waveform, the interpreting physician may mistake the data as true information, which could lead to a misdiagnosis. Aliasing is considered an artifact that demonstrates an error in imaging because the waveform tends to wrap around the baseline. There are many steps that can be taken to eliminate signals that display aliasing. The first step a sonographer should try is to adjust the pulse repetition frequency (PRF) (velocity scale). In arteries, the blood flow is moving rapidly so increasing the PRF may help unwrap the spectral display. This step increases the Nyquist limit, which is also known as the aliasing frequency and is equal to half of the PRF. If this alone does not take care of aliasing, the baseline may be adjusted accordingly. Another helpful tip to eliminate aliasing is to switch to a lower frequency transducer or even find a window that is at a more shallow location. The angle of incidence could also be increased to help eliminate aliasing. If that still doesn't work, then the user could switch to continuous-wave Doppler.

Operator Controls Affecting Frame Rate

Many of the parameters that a sonographer can adjust will have an effect on the frame rate. The frame rate controls temporal resolution, which is the ability of the system to accurately track the location of structures with regard to time. If a system tends to "lag" or have a low frame rate, this will result in poor temporal resolution. Temporal resolution is considered optimal when there are several frames per second. Controls that a sonographer can alter to affect frame rate include changing the scanning depth. If a system is imaging a structure that is deep in the body, the temporal resolution will be poorer because there is more listening time, which results in a lower frame rate. Changes that the sonographer can make to alter the number of pulses sent into the body are changing the number of focal zones, adjusting the field of view (sector size), and changing the line density.

Multiple Focal Zones

Modern imaging systems have the capability to operate while using multiple focal zones. Using multiple foci will greatly improve the detail of an image, but users must balance detail and the time required for the study. If a sonographer is looking at an object using a single focus, the temporal resolution will be superior because the frame rate is higher. If additional focal zones are added, not only are more pulses required, but extra pulses are also needed in each scan line. This will degrade the temporal resolution because the frame rate is slower. A multifocus sound beam will greatly

Copyright © Mometrix Media. You have been licensed one copy of this document for personal use only. Any other reproduction or redistribution is strictly prohibited. All rights reserved.
This content is provided for test preparation purposes only and does not imply an endorsement by Mometrix of any particular political, scientific, or religious point of view.

improve the lateral resolution of an image because the beam is narrowed over many depths, but the temporal resolution will suffer.

Persistence

Persistence is an averaging technique that will combine images from older frames with those of newer data. In gray-scale imaging, persistence can be used to smooth out an image or reduce the amount of noise present. Persistence is also found to be useful in color Doppler imaging, especially if the vessels to be visualized are deeper in the body, to identify vessels that contain slow-moving blood, or if there is an obstruction of a vessel. Smaller vessels can also be identified more readily than with methods that do not implement persistence. Users should know that the temporal resolution is often decreased when persistence is applied to an image.

Interrogating a Vessel Displaying Slow Flow

PRF stands for pulse repetition frequency, but it is also referred to as the scale while pulsed Doppler is being used. In this example, the vessel being interrogated displays blood flow that is moving slowly. If color is not optimized after turning on color Doppler, the sonographer would decrease the PRF so that the ultrasound system is more receptive in picking up slower blood flow signals. Blood that is within the venous portion of the circulatory system is often where slow flow will be visualized. If this step alone does not improve color Doppler visualization of the vessel, the sonographer may need to increase the color gain. If the operator chooses to increase the PRF scale, he or she may notice a decreased sensitivity to slow flow states. However, if one is interrogating a vessel with higher velocity flow, the PRF should be set higher in order to raise the Nyquist limit and prevent or eliminate aliasing.

Copyright © Mometrix Media. You have been licensed one copy of this document for personal use only. Any other reproduction or redistribution is strictly prohibited. All rights reserved.
This content is provided for test preparation purposes only and does not imply an endorsement by Mometrix of any particular political, scientific, or religious point of view.

Image Formation

Relationship of PZT Diameter and Frequency

The diameter of the lead zirconate titanate (PZT) crystal does not contribute to the frequency of the sound wave transmitted by the transducer. The crystal in an ultrasound transducer is referred to as the active element or PZT crystal. Companies that construct ultrasound probes use PZT material that is of assorted thickness in order to offer customers transducers with different frequencies. Vascular technologists should be aware that the frequency of the sound wave is inversely related to the thickness of the active element (PZT crystal). Crystals that are thinner provide the sonographer with pulses that are shorter at higher frequencies. PZT elements that are thicker allow for a longer wavelength and lower frequency. For diagnostic probes, the thickness of the active element is 0.2–1 mm.

Transducer Used During a Transcranial Study

Vascular technologists must choose a transducer that is high powered and capable of penetrating the patient's skull. When performing a transcranial study, multiple windows will be used so more power is required. Whether the method used will be transcranial Doppler (TCD) or transcranial Doppler imaging (TCDI), the transducer will be one of low frequency. TCD uses pulsed-wave, nonimaging transducers that are 1–3 MHz that will provide important information regarding how deep the vessel being interrogating is and the direction of blood flowing within the vessel. Other factors that can be measured are the PSV and EDV. TCDI transducers are between 2 and 3 MHz and are part of a traditional ultrasound system that uses phased-array transducers. TCDI systems have calculation packages for PSV and EDV.

Frequency of Ultrasound Transducers

The frequency of ultrasound transducers relies on how the active element is activated. These can either be determined by continuous- or pulsed-wave principles. Pulsed-wave ultrasound will send short electrical impulses that travel from the system to excite the PZT element in the probe. In contrast, ultrasound transducers that are considered to be continuous wave tend to steadily induce an electrical impulse that activates the probe's active element. The following equation can be used to formulate the frequency: $electrical\ frequency = acoustic\ frequency$.

Sample

While using a continuous-wave transducer, if the voltage is 14 MHz, what is the frequency of the sound beam?

If the voltage is 14 MHz, this is the electrical frequency. Therefore, the frequency of the sound beam would also be 14 MHz.

Sample

If a 10 MHz transducer can be bumped up to 12 MHz and lowered to 8 MHz, what will the main frequency be?

The main frequency of a transducer is the frequency that is being emitted from the probe into the body of the patient. Modern technology enables users to easily change the frequency without switching probes. In the above example, the main frequency (also known as the resonant frequency) is 10 MHz. However, the range of frequencies transmitted is 8 MHz to 12 MHz. The bandwidth can also be determined from this example. Bandwidth refers to the frequency range within a sound beam. This can be calculated by subtracting the lowest possible frequency from the

Copyright © Mometrix Media. You have been licensed one copy of this document for personal use only. Any other reproduction or redistribution is strictly prohibited. All rights reserved.
This content is provided for test preparation purposes only and does not imply an endorsement by Mometrix of any particular political, scientific, or religious point of view.

highest available frequency. In this case, the bandwidth would be $12 - 8 = 4$ MHz. Because imaging transducers can produce many frequencies, they tend to have a wide bandwidth.

Fundamental Frequency vs. Harmonic Frequency

The fundamental frequency is the actual frequency that is being imparted from the ultrasound transducer and passed into the patient. This is also known as the transmitted frequency. Sometimes, the ultrasound beam is altered and creates exams that are not of diagnostic quality. Modern ultrasound systems offer harmonic imaging to help increase diagnostic confidence in those difficult studies. If a sonographer uses harmonic ultrasound, the harmonic frequency used is two times higher than the fundamental (transmitted) frequency. The sound beam is altered less, and the harmonic ultrasound beam helps improve diagnostic capabilities. Tissue and contrast harmonics are two examples of the types of harmonic ultrasound in use today.

Imaging and Nonimaging Transducer Design

One of the main differences in transducer design for imaging and nonimaging transducers is that imaging transducers contain a layer called backing material. This is used to create short pulses by inhibiting the amount of time that the PZT crystals are vibrating. Remember that short pulses create diagnostic-quality images, but the layer of backing material tends to lessen the sensitivity. Nonimaging transducers do not contain this backing material; therefore, they either produce a wave that is continuous, or they tend to have very long pulses. Neither of these two types will be effective in producing an ultrasound image. Probes that are capable of producing diagnostic-quality exams are referred to as being of a low quality factor (Q-factor), and they have a wide bandwidth.

Relationship Between Q-Factor and Pulse Duration/Length

Nonimaging transducers are not capable of producing an ultrasound image. Examples of nonimaging transducers are continuous-wave Doppler, which can be used to determine blood flow. Therapeutic ultrasound is another application that doesn't provide an image during use. These transducers do not contain backing material; therefore, they create long pulses. Long pulses, as in this situation, refer to the length of the pulse as well as the amount of time the crystal is excited. The lack of backing material also allows smaller reflectors to be converted more easily into electrical signals as they return to the transducer. Nonimaging transducers are considered to have a high Q-factor because the bandwidth tends to be narrow.

Advantages Linear Phased-Array Transducer

There are many advantages of using any transducer with phased-array technology. For example, the sonographer can electronically focus the ultrasound beam at all depths during an exam. This allows the operator to customize the ultrasound system's settings based on what is required. Focusing can be optimized regardless of the depth of the anatomical structure being interrogated. Steering is also controlled electronically. With linear sequential phased-array transducers, the part that touches the patient is flat, but the beam is sent into the body in a nonlinear fashion. In other words, the pulses can also reach structures in the body that are not directly in front of them. Linear sequential phased-array probes have very small footprints. This is great for cardiac or pediatric scanning when the user is attempting to image via the intercostal spaces.

Monitoring the TI During an Ultrasound Exam

Ultrasound should only be used for clinical exams in which the benefits outweigh the risks. One risk during an exam is an elevation of temperature in tissues exposed to the ultrasound beam. The sonographer should already know that the TI will be highest during an exam with a high-frequency, high-intensity beam. This heating depends on the exposure time and temperature. Typically, the greatest increase in temperature is witnessed with spectral Doppler exams. Pulsed-wave Doppler

Copyright © Mometrix Media. You have been licensed one copy of this document for personal use only. Any other reproduction or redistribution is strictly prohibited. All rights reserved.
This content is provided for test preparation purposes only and does not imply an endorsement by Mometrix of any particular political, scientific, or religious point of view.

requires more energy than does B-mode or gray-scale imaging. Ideally, the TI should be 1.0 or less and the time should be minimized to prevent tissue heating. If the TI is 1.0, there is a possibility that the temperature of the tissue will increase by 1 degree. TI is expressed by TIS, TIB, and TIC.

Focusing Techniques for Ultrasound Transducers

There are various techniques used to focus an ultrasound beam. Focusing is a method that is used to improve resolution of an ultrasound image by creating a sound beam that is narrow. External focusing using a lens is one way to improve lateral resolution. This is an example of a fixed-focusing or conventional method in which a lens is embedded in front of the active element, which will provide a narrow beam in the region of focus. A more common method of fixed focusing that does not need a lens is internal focusing. This form includes a crystal that has a curved shape, but it also results in an ultrasound beam that is tapered. Electronic focusing by using phased-array technology allows the sonographer to adjust the focus. This is only available on probes that have many PZT crystals.

Fraunhofer Zone

Vascular technologists should be aware that the shape and width of the ultrasound beam changes as it moves. The Fraunhofer zone is also referred to as the far zone, which is the area of the sound beam located distal to (beyond) the focus. The focus is the area of the beam in which much of the energy is concentrated because the beam is the narrowest. At the focal point (focus) the diameter of the ultrasound beam is half of the diameter of the transducer. This includes the proximal (beginning) of the Fraunhofer zone, which is close to the focus. At the end of the far zone, however, the beam diverges to the same diameter of the transducer once again. The end of the far zone is often referred to as two focal depths.

Focusing Has on the Ultrasound Beam

When a sonographer applies focusing during an exam, many changes take place within the ultrasound beam. Remember that focusing is used to optimize the lateral resolution of the exam. When focusing is used, the energy of the beam is concentrated into one small area (focus), thus improving the lateral resolution. An ultrasound beam that is focused will create a focal zone that is more compact than a beam that is not focused. A focused beam also tends to move the focal point closer to the face of the probe being used. This will result in a near zone that is shorter when compared to an unfocused beam. Although the ultrasound beam's shape changes, the width is also changed. The beam's diameter will diverge in the far field, but it tends to be smaller in the near zone with the smallest possible component at the focus.

Near Field

Sonographers should be aware that the shape and width of the ultrasound beam change as it moves. The near zone is also known as the Fresnel zone and is the area located between the transducer and the focus. The diameter of the beam is the narrowest at the focus, which is at the distal portion of the near field; therefore, the beam gradually tapers as it gets closer to the focus. The width of the ultrasound beam near the transducer will be equal to the transducer diameter. At the focus, the width of the ultrasound beam is equal to half of the beam diameter. The length of the near zone is also known as the focal depth and is the region from the transducer to the focus.

Beam Diameter at the Proximal Portion of the Far Field

Vascular technologists should be aware that the far field (the Fraunhofer zone) is the region that is beyond the focus. The proximal portion of the far field is the area that is located closest to the focus. In fact, half of the focal zone includes this proximal portion of the far field, and it is where the ultrasound beam is most narrow. This is the region that offers the best image detail, and the images

Copyright © Mometrix Media. You have been licensed one copy of this document for personal use only. Any other reproduction or redistribution is strictly prohibited. All rights reserved.
This content is provided for test preparation purposes only and does not imply an endorsement by Mometrix of any particular political, scientific, or religious point of view.

that result at this depth are more accurately portrayed than other imaging depths. The beam tends to taper at the focus and, therefore, at the proximal portion of the far field. In this area, the beam is half as wide as the diameter of the transducer and offers the greatest amount of detail.

Time of Flight

Ultrasound systems can determine the depth of an object by calculating the time of flight. This time refers to having the transducer send out a pulse, and once the reflector has been identified, the signal is returned back to the transducer. The round trip of the pulse is calculated by the range equation and allows for a very precise calculation: $d = \frac{1}{2}ct$, where d is the depth, c is the speed of sound in soft tissue, and t is the time of flight. The ultrasound system is designed to recognize the speed of sound in soft tissue as 1540 m/s (1.54 mm/μs). Sonographers should realize that the time of flight is directly associated with the depth. If an object being imaged is shallow, the time of flight is short. Conversely, if the reflector is deeper in location, the time of flight is greater.

Effect of Distance on Attenuation

Attenuation is measured in decibels and is defined as a decrease in amplitude, power, and intensity as sound travels in the body. In soft tissue, two components that influence attenuation are the distance traveled and the frequency of the ultrasound beam. There is a direct correlation between attenuation and the distance that the sound beam navigates. There is a direct relationship between the frequency of the beam and attenuation. In other words, sound beams that are required to travel a longer distance will demonstrate greater amounts of attenuation and become weaker. Using higher frequencies will also cause greater attenuation of the ultrasound beam. A sound beam that travels a short distance will have a smaller degree of attenuation and a beam that is stronger. Lower frequency transducers will create a beam with less attenuation.

Effect of Imaging Depth on the Frame Rate

Frame rate refers to the capability of an ultrasound system to produce multiple frames per second. The temporal resolution is how precisely an object in motion is portrayed from one second to the next and is decided by the frame rate. The frame rate depends on the imaging depth because a reflector that is deeper in the body will result in a longer time of flight to return back to the transducer. A structure that is deeper in the body results in a lower frame rate, which tends to degrade the temporal resolution. If a structure is located more superficially or shallowly, the time of flight is shorter, which results in a higher frame rate and improved temporal resolution. Depth can be controlled by the ultrasound user.

Avoiding Range Ambiguity

Range ambiguity is an imaging error in which echoes have not yet returned to the transducer before the transmission of the next pulse. If the PRF is too high while scanning a structure deep in the body, range ambiguity may occur. If this happens, the system will incorrectly place the received reflections closer to the probe than their actual depth. Keep in mind that the PRF represents the number of pulses sent into the body every second and is presented in units of hertz (Hz). The normal range of PRF or imaging systems is 1,000–10,000 Hz. If a sonographer increases the imaging depth, the system automatically decreases the PRF in order to avoid range ambiguity. In other words, the PRF is inversely related to the imaging depth so if the scan depth is twice as deep, the ultrasound system will automatically reduce the PRF by half.

Effect of Changing the Depth on the PRP

Vascular technologists are familiar with the fact that the pulse repetition period (PRP) consists of the time that the pulse is on (send) and the off time (listening) as pulses are sent out of the

Copyright © Mometrix Media. You have been licensed one copy of this document for personal use only. Any other reproduction or redistribution is strictly prohibited. All rights reserved.
This content is provided for test preparation purposes only and does not imply an endorsement by Mometrix of any particular political, scientific, or religious point of view.

transducer. There is a direct relationship between the scanning depth and the PRP. If a sonographer is attempting to scan an object located deep in the body, there will be more listening (receive) time and a lower PRF. If the reflector being examined happens to be shallower, the PRP is shorter because the listening time is decreased. Sonographers can, of course, change the imaging depth with a control on the ultrasound system. Keep in mind that the PRP and PRF are reciprocals of each other and have an inverse relationship.

13 μs Rule

Ultrasound machines are designed to calculate the speed of the ultrasound wave in soft tissue as 1.54 mm/μs. The time of flight refers to the time it takes for a pulse to leave the transducer, hit a reflector, and return back to the transducer. The depth of the reflector can be calculated as being 1 cm when the time of flight equals 13 μs. Using this rule, if a target is 2 cm deep, the time of flight will be twice as long, equating to 26 μs. If the time of flight is 39 μs, the depth of the reflector will be 3 cm. The vascular technologist should be aware of the reflector depth and the total distance traveled. For example, if a question states that the time of flight was 13 μs and it is asked what the *total* distance traveled is, the answer would be 2 cm. At 13 μs, the depth would only be 1 cm, but the total distance (including the return trip) would be 1 cm + 1 cm = 2 cm.

Corrective Action If Aliasing Is Visualized

Sonographers are aware of the many steps that can be taken to eliminate aliasing, but sometimes the actual depth of the anatomical structure is more of an issue than the settings on the machine. If an operator has adjusted the PRF scale and the baseline to no avail, considering the depth of the reflector is yet another option. The operator can try to find a different window that still allows the structures to be seen while placing the anatomical structures at a more superficial location. This corrective action can eliminate aliasing because when moving from a deeper to a more superficial location, the PRF is increased, which in turn raises the Nyquist limit.

Attenuation

Attenuation is the reduction of the intensity of the ultrasound beam as it passes through tissue. More attenuation occurs when the beam travels a greater distance in the body. Echoes that return from a shallower location in the body will tend to be stronger than those that are located deeper. In order for the sonographer to compensate for the amount of attenuation within tissues, the time gain compensation (TGC) or depth gain compensation can be adjusted. This control will typically appear as slide pods that can be adjusted. Each level represents different depths within the body. The overall goal of TGC is to create an image that demonstrates uniform brightness from the top of the display to the bottom.

Adjusting for Echoes

Vascular technologists can visualize the depth of every reflector because there will be a scale on one side of the image that correlates to how deep they are located within the body. Every dot typically represents 1 cm. The ultrasound user can count down 4 cm from the top to locate the reflector that is appearing too bright on the ultrasound screen. In order to adjust for the increased echogenicity of the structure, the sonographer can find the TGC slide pod that correlates to that location and move the slider to the user's left (or toward the right of the ultrasound system). TCG can be used in conjunction with receiver gain (amplification) to provide an image that has a consistent brightness throughout the image.

Regions of a TGC Curve

A TGC curve has an *x*-axis as well as a *y*-axis. The horizontal *x*-axis refers to how much compensation is necessary for the depth of the object being imaged (*y*-axis). The top of the *y*-axis

Copyright © Mometrix Media. You have been licensed one copy of this document for personal use only. Any other reproduction or redistribution is strictly prohibited. All rights reserved.
This content is provided for test preparation purposes only and does not imply an endorsement by Mometrix of any particular political, scientific, or religious point of view.

represents the patient's skin, and as it moves down it refers to tissues that are located deeper in the body. The near gain is located superficially near the skin's surface. At this location, the structures being imaged need very little TGC because not much attenuation occurs. The slope is the middle portion of the TGC curve in which more compensation is necessary because of the greater depths. The knee is located at the distal portion of the slope and is where the most compensation will occur. The region of the far gain is distal to the knee at an ever-greater depth that also designates that the greatest amount of compensation has been offered by the machine.

AMPLIFICATION

Amplification refers to the brightness of the ultrasound signal. Amplification can be measured in decibels (dB). Compensation is a type of amplification, so it is also measured in decibels. Amplification is the first process that takes place in the receiver. It will differentiate the strength of the beam as it enters and exits the receiver of the ultrasound system. The normal range for amplification of an image ranges from 60–100 dB. Changing only the amplification is not enough to create an image that is the same level of brightness throughout. The user must also consider adjusting the compensation. Compensation is the second process in the receiver and can be used in conjunction with amplification to create an image that demonstrates uniform brightness.

CHANGING THE OVERALL RECEIVER GAIN

When a sonographer changes the overall receiver gain on an ultrasound system, it is the amplification that is being increased or decreased. This action takes place in the receiver and has a uniform effect on the image by changing the strength of the voltages that the probe has produced. If the receiver gain is increased, a brighter image will appear throughout the entire image. If the receiver gain is decreased, the overall image becomes darker. Unlike output power, if the gain is increased, the signal-to-noise ratio is not changed. An increase in power will enhance the signal-to-noise ratio.

MAKING THE ENTIRE IMAGE BRIGHTER

Sonographers should always keep the as low as reasonably achievable (ALARA) principle in mind during all diagnostic imaging exams. This principle is one that is practiced to reduce the possibility of adverse effects during an ultrasound exam. A sonographer may make an entire image brighter by increasing the output power, but this will also increase the voltage exposure to the patient. If the output power is increased, more voltage is applied to the transducer, which increases the strength of the pulse sent into the body. A safer alternative to increase the brightness of the entire image is to increase the gain, which does not expose the patient to more powerful voltages.

MAKING THE ENTIRE IMAGE DARKER

Vascular technologists should always keep the ALARA principle in mind during all diagnostic imaging exams. This principle is followed in order to reduce the possibility of bioeffects during an ultrasound exam. Two controls on the machine will make an entire image darker or brighter as the result of adjusting the knob. If the entire image is too bright and the user wants to darken it, the amount of receiver gain may be decreased in order to darken the image. However, this is not the best step to take in order to demonstrate knowledge of the ALARA principle. Receiver gain will allow an image to become darker (or brighter) but using this control does not affect the exposure to the patient. If one needs to darken an image while lessening patient exposure, the output (acoustic) power should be decreased. This will result in less patient exposure because the strength of the voltage applied to the PZT crystals is weaker.

Copyright © Mometrix Media. You have been licensed one copy of this document for personal use only. Any other reproduction or redistribution is strictly prohibited. All rights reserved.
This content is provided for test preparation purposes only and does not imply an endorsement by Mometrix of any particular political, scientific, or religious point of view.

Applying Multiple Foci on the Temporal Resolution and Frame Rate

If an ultrasound user applies multiple focal zones during an exam, the temporal resolution degrades because this action tends to slow down the frame rate. Compared to using just one focal zone, each additional focal zone that is used requires the system to produce more pulses throughout each scan line, which, in turn, increases the time necessary to produce every single image. This will, however, improve the lateral resolution to more accurately display the reflectors because the beam is tighter within the focal regions. It is up to the sonographer to decide which type of resolution will better aid in getting the correct diagnosis for the patient.

Improvement of Lateral Resolution

It is important to realize that lateral resolution is improved with sound beams that are narrower. The shape of the ultrasound beam tends to change regarding the depth; therefore, the lateral resolution tends to be improved upon at depths at which the sound beam is narrow. This depth is at the focus, and when multiple focal points are used the beam becomes tapered over a greater imaging depth, which greatly enhances the accuracy of the images that are produced. It is important to remember that although the lateral resolution is improved when multiple focal zones are used, the temporal resolution tends to decline because more time is necessary to produce the image.

Spectral Display Showing Too Much Noise

A vascular technologist should be aware of various spectral Doppler artifacts so that the results are not misconstrued. The parameters on the ultrasound machine should be understood and set correctly so that information is not lost or added to the image. Noise is one such artifact that can degrade the quality of the spectral waveform. Noise can typically be identified easily by the user and can be alleviated by reducing the amount of the pulsed Doppler gain. Noise may appear similar to spectral broadening, and one would not want the interpreting physician to incorrectly diagnose it as turbulent flow. The user should turn down the gain so that the spectral window is clear, but the systolic and diastolic components can easily be visualized along with forward flow patterns.

Adjusting the Spectral Doppler Gain If Display Is Hard to Visualize

Pulsed-wave Doppler provides important information that can be used to diagnose many disorders in patients. Correct Doppler settings are crucial, and vascular technologists must have a strong understanding of not only anatomy, but also ultrasound physics. If the machine is not set properly, an artifact can occur that may limit the amount of diagnostic information present. If the sonographer turns on the pulsed-wave Doppler, but the spectral display can barely be visualized, then the next step will be to turn up the pulsed-wave Doppler's gain. It is important to note that if the gain is turned up too high, noise may appear in the spectral display. One can increase the gain by turning up the gain until noise appears. At this point, slowly reduce the gain until the noise disappears.

Correcting Multiple Speckled Colors

If a vascular technologist visualizes multiple speckled colors throughout the color box after turning on color Doppler, the first step to correct this noise is to turn the color gain down. Color gain that is set correctly is adjusted so that the amplitude is set at the highest level without displaying color speckles. Aliasing, color Doppler gain that is set too high, and turbulent flow all have a different appearance, so ultrasound users should be able to discern what is taking place. Some are artifacts and can be corrected with the adjustment of parameters on the ultrasound machine.

Copyright © Mometrix Media. You have been licensed one copy of this document for personal use only. Any other reproduction or redistribution is strictly prohibited. All rights reserved.
This content is provided for test preparation purposes only and does not imply an endorsement by Mometrix of any particular political, scientific, or religious point of view.

Optimizing Color Flow of a Patent Carotid Artery

If a vascular technologist cannot visualize color during a carotid duplex exam, the first thing to do is to determine the angle of the color box with the direction of blood flow. It is important for sonographers to remember that if the color box is perpendicular (at a 90-degree angle) to a vessel, color will never be visualized. Modern systems allow color boxes to be steered with linear transducers, which will prevent the beam from being perpendicular to the vessel. Next, the user can increase the color gain. This demonstrates the amplification of signals within blood vessels, but it will not show blood flow if it is not actually present. The velocity scale is also important to adjust if blood flow is not well demonstrated or if aliasing occurs.

Doppler Angle

In order for the vascular technologist to obtain the most accurate measurement during a carotid duplex exam, the moving red blood cells should be located parallel to the transducer. In this case, the measurement reflects the velocity located in all parts of the ultrasound wave. A positive Doppler frequency occurs when the velocity of the returning signals from blood cells moving towards the transducer is greater than the transmitted velocity. When the blood is not moving exactly parallel to the sound beam, the velocity that is taken will be a value that is not as accurate. For example, if the angle cursor is larger than the actual Doppler angle, the velocity will be too high. If the angle cursor is lower than the angle that is parallel to the vessel wall, then the velocity will be underestimated.

Doppler Equation

When a sonographer is using routine gray-scale ultrasound imaging, the ideal incident beam is when the transducer is placed 90 degrees to the object being scanned. For Doppler, however, the maximum frequency shift will be obtained with an incident angle of either 0 degrees (blood flow moving toward the transducer) or 180 degrees (blood cells moving away from the transducer). By using the Doppler equation, the cosine of 90 degrees is equal to 0, so we cannot measure any Doppler frequency when the incident beam is 90 degrees (perpendicular) to the direction of blood flow.

Range Resolution

Pulsed-wave Doppler provides range resolution, which provides users with the ability to know precisely where the velocity measurements are being taken. When pulsed-wave Doppler is selected on the machine, the user will move the gate to the blood vessel to be interrogated. The size of the gate, also known as the sample volume, can be adjusted so that the user is sampling a good portion of the blood vessel. Sometimes, the vascular technologist will notice that blood flow from arteries and veins is displayed. If this happens, the user can adjust the size of the gate in order to obtain data only from the vessel of interest. One may also have to adjust the location because perhaps the gate was accidently moved into a different vessel. Modern systems will have a triplex function that allows the user to display gray-scale, color, and spectral Doppler at the same time. If you are picking up flow from two different vessels, update the triplex image and move the sample volume into the vessel that you want to investigate.

Wall Filter

Role in Color Doppler During a Vascular Exam

The wall filter is an important tool that vascular technologists can use to remove Doppler shifts below a certain set frequency during spectral and color Doppler interrogations. In other words, this control will help remove the lower frequency Doppler signals that may arise from motion that anatomical structures such as the heart or blood vessels create. Wall filters are also referred to as

Copyright © Mometrix Media. You have been licensed one copy of this document for personal use only. Any other reproduction or redistribution is strictly prohibited. All rights reserved.
This content is provided for test preparation purposes only and does not imply an endorsement by Mometrix of any particular political, scientific, or religious point of view.

high-pass filters, and they do not play a role in higher Doppler shifts such as those created from the movement of blood cells in the circulatory system. Sonographers should remember that blood that is moving slower will create a lower frequency Doppler shift. The system is less likely to detect blood that is moving slowly when the wall filter is set at a higher level.

Effect of Increasing Wall Filter on Low-Velocity Blood Flow

If an ultrasound user increases the wall filter while using color Doppler, this will only affect the low-velocity flow in vessels. If a sonographer has an image in which the blood flow can be seen with color Doppler in an artery and a vein, but increases the wall filter setting high enough, the arterial flow will be the only one visualized. Venous blood flow is slower than arterial, and by changing the wall filter (the high-pass filter) to a setting that is high, it removes or rejects the color Doppler from the vein. However, the wall filter will not affect vessels in which high-velocity flow occurs. It may, however, eliminate any ghosting artifacts, which appear as color Doppler that is visualized on the outside lumen of the vessel due to the motion created by a pulsating blood vessel.

Effect of Increasing Wall Filter on Lower Velocity Flows

Vascular technologists should be aware that increasing the wall filter during spectral analysis will only effectively remove the lower frequency Doppler shifts from slower blood flow. On a spectral Doppler waveform, lower frequency shifts are visualized near the baseline, so this is where the elimination will take place. This will not affect the vascular technologist's ability to measure high-velocity flows. It is important to remember that a high-wall filter level will decrease the ability to detect slower flow. During a carotid Doppler study, if the user cannot measure the velocity of the end-diastolic flow, it would be beneficial to decrease the wall filter setting.

Factors Increasing/Reducing the Frame Rate During an Ultrasound

Vascular technologists are acutely aware of factors that will either increase or reduce the frame rate during an ultrasound exam. If the frame rate is low, it takes longer to create an image and a lag may be visualized in the image. Temporal resolution is the ability of the ultrasound system to track reflectors from one second to the next. When the frame rate is high, the temporal resolution is good. If the frame rate is low, the temporal resolution suffers because fewer frames are created every second. There is a direct relationship between the scanning depth and the temporal resolution. The PRF is not a button or knob on the machine that can be adjusted. Sonographers should recall that the PRF is adjusted when the scanning depth is changed and will notice an indirect relationship. If the depth of view is increased, the PRF will be lower. If the depth of view is shallow, then the PRF will be higher. In this example, the PRF is lower, which means that the object being examined is deeper in the body. A greater depth will result in a decrease of the temporal resolution.

Visualize Flow That Moves Rapidly in Vessels

Correct optimization of color flow is always the goal when examining vessels while using color Doppler. In order to get the entire vessel to fill in properly, one of the first steps the sonographer can perform after turning on the color flow is to adjust the PRF. The PRF is often referred to as the color scale when color Doppler is activated. In this example, the blood flow is moving at a rapid pace, and it is likely an artery, so the ultrasound user would want to increase the PRF. This raises the Nyquist limit of the machine, which will help avoid aliasing. Aliasing can occur in color Doppler imaging and will appear as a variety of colors within the lumen of the blood vessel. The next step is to increase the color gain if the vessel is not completely filled with color.

Eliminating Signals That Display Aliasing

Aliasing is considered an artifact that demonstrates an error in imaging. The vascular technologist has several options to eliminate signals that display aliasing. The first parameter a sonographer

Copyright © Mometrix Media. You have been licensed one copy of this document for personal use only. Any other reproduction or redistribution is strictly prohibited. All rights reserved.
This content is provided for test preparation purposes only and does not imply an endorsement by Mometrix of any particular political, scientific, or religious point of view.

should try to adjust is the PRF (velocity scale). Because this is an artery, the blood flow is moving rapidly so increasing the PRF may help unwrap the spectral display. This step increases the Nyquist limit, which is also known as the aliasing frequency and is equal to half the PRF. If this alone does not take care of aliasing, the baseline may be adjusted accordingly. Another helpful tip to eliminate aliasing is to switch to a lower frequency transducer or even to find a window that is at a shallower location. The angle of incidence could also be increased to help eliminate aliasing.

Maximizing Scale to Prevent Aliasing

Many parameters can be controlled by the sonographer to prevent aliasing during an exam. One of these is to change the PRF scale. Remember that aliasing occurs if the measured frequency shift is greater than the Nyquist limit. The Nyquist limit is equal to half of the PRF. If the PRF is adjusted to the highest possible level, the Nyquist limit will also be higher, so aliasing is not as likely to occur. However, with extremely high-velocity blood flow, even if the PRF is maximized aliasing may still occur. If it does, the sonographer could switch to continuous-wave Doppler because aliasing does not take place when it is used. Users should be aware that when maximizing the PRF scale, the system may not recognize vessels with slower blood flow.

Angle of the Color Box

If color is not displayed within a vessel after turning on color Doppler, the sonographer should immediately consider the angle of the incident beam in regard to the flow angle. If the incident beam is 90 degrees to the blood vessel being interrogated, color will not be visualized. According to the Doppler equation, the cosine of 90 is zero; therefore, no color can be visualized. The next thing that a sonographer can do to improve visualization of color Doppler is to angle the color box so the incident beam is not 90 degrees. The ultrasound user can also increase the scale and the color gain in order to increase the amount of blood visualized in the vessel.

Size and Location of the Color Box

Vascular technologists can adjust many controls on the ultrasound system pertaining to the use of color Doppler and frame rate during an exam. In order to optimize the temporal resolution, the user needs to be aware of the size and location of the color box. The color box will allow the velocity information to be portrayed as an overlay of color on the traditional gray-scale image. As the color box size increases, the frame rate or temporal resolution decreases because more information needs to be processed. This is especially important when considering the width of the color box. More scan lines are required with a wider color box, and more time is required by the system to process the acquired data. The sonographer should limit the size of the color box to the anatomy of interest. The location is also something to consider because a deeper location may actually produce aliasing of the color flow because the PRF is lower.

Discerning the Direction of Blood Flow

While Using a Linear Probe When Steering Is Used

Vascular technologists should check the color map on the image to determine which colors represent the toward (above the baseline) and away (beneath the baseline) flow in a blood vessel. When the color box is angled, instead of a rectangle it is in the shape of a parallelogram. Users must find a landmark that can be thought of as the pretend location of the probe within the vessel. In order to do this, find the top corner of the steered color box and draw a line down. The imaginary line that does not bump into any other portion of the color box will be where the fictional probe is located. From the placement of the probe, determine if the color within the box is moving toward or away. The direction of blood flow is decided as the user tracks either to or from the position of the transducer. This will either be a left-to-right or right-to-left movement.

Copyright © Mometrix Media. You have been licensed one copy of this document for personal use only. Any other reproduction or redistribution is strictly prohibited. All rights reserved.
This content is provided for test preparation purposes only and does not imply an endorsement by Mometrix of any particular political, scientific, or religious point of view.

Relation of Contrast to Dynamic Range

The dynamic range is a ratio between the largest to smallest of intensities that can accurately be displayed by the ultrasound system. The units of dynamic range are decibels. If an ultrasound machine produces an image that displays numerous shades of gray (which contains more information), the image would be considered to have a wide dynamic range. An image with numerous shades of gray demonstrated is classified as demonstrating low contrast. On the other hand, if the system produces an image that is considered to have a narrow dynamic range, it will tend to be more black and white and will have fewer shades of gray. The end result of a narrow dynamic range is a high-contrast image.

Modifying the Dynamic Range by Adjusting Compression on the Ultrasound System

Compression is a parameter on the ultrasound system that allows the vascular technologist to change the number of shades of gray that are available to produce an image that is visually appealing. The purpose of using this button is to produce an image that contains as much data as possible to make a diagnosis without producing an image that is particularly dark or overly gray. Dynamic range is another name for compression, and it has a greater effect on the signals that are weaker and has a reduced effect on the reflections that are stronger. If the end user prefers an image having a smoother appearance, then a wider range (numerous shades of gray) would be preferred.

Optimizing the Temporal Resolution by Decreasing the Width of the Sector

Vascular technologists are aware that a high frame rate is ideal during an exam. If the ultrasound user would like to optimize the temporal resolution during an exam, the depth should be decreased. However, if additional steps needed to be taken to further improve (increase) the frame rate, the operator could decrease the field of view (the width of the sector). When the field of view is smaller, there are fewer pulses necessary to create the image, which takes less time. The frame rate (temporal resolution) is inversely proportional to the sector size of the image. Some anatomical areas can fit in a smaller sector size, especially when imaging in the transverse plane, so this is one step that can quickly be taken to improve the temporal resolution. Also, being cognizant of how many focal zones are being used is another step that can be taken because reducing the amount of focusing may also improve the temporal resolution.

Eliminate Aliasing by Adjusting the Baseline

During a spectral display, the system can document flow that is moving in opposite directions. Flow that is visualized above the baseline demonstrates blood flow that is moving toward the transducer. Flow below the baseline signifies blood flow traveling away from the transducer. If the user notices that flow is wrapping around the baseline, this is an aliasing artifact. Sonographers can take many steps to eliminate aliasing. One such corrective measure is to adjust the baseline. If the flow is above the baseline, but aliasing occurs, the user can move the baseline lower so that the entire waveform is going in one direction. This allows for extremely high-velocity flow to be shown moving in the correct direction and still allows for an accurate measurement.

Calculating the Acceleration Time

It can be helpful to calculate the acceleration time during an arterial study to discern if the patient's symptoms are due to inflow or outflow conditions. If an obstruction of the artery is present in the region of the blood vessel that is proximal to where the vascular technologist has the transducer, there will be a longer amount of time between the start of systole and the greatest peak velocity. On the other hand, the acceleration time will not be longer if the patient has a significant stenosis or

Copyright © Mometrix Media. You have been licensed one copy of this document for personal use only. Any other reproduction or redistribution is strictly prohibited. All rights reserved.
This content is provided for test preparation purposes only and does not imply an endorsement by Mometrix of any particular political, scientific, or religious point of view.

occlusion in the region of the artery that is in a more distal location to where the artery is being interrogated. Notably, an example of inflow disease would be an aortoiliac stenosis because it refers to problems of blood traveling into the legs from the heart. An example of outflow disease would be a stenosis because blood is attempting to travel from the femoral artery to the rest of the lower extremity.

SAMPLE

If the acceleration time of the CFA was calculated to be 145 ms, explain why this is considered to be an abnormal finding.

When evaluating the acceleration time of the CFA, it is considered to be abnormal if this number is greater than or equal to 133 msec. Because 145 ms is greater than 133, the acceleration time of this particular patient is abnormal, which correlates to significant disease of the iliac artery. To gain a better understanding of an abnormal finding, it is also important to study the appearance of the arterial waveform. The acceleration time is considered to be abnormal if there is a slow upslope from the beginning of systole to the maximum peak velocity. When there is a rapid upslope demonstrated from the beginning of systole to the maximum peak velocity, the acceleration time is considered to be normal.

Copyright © Mometrix Media. You have been licensed one copy of this document for personal use only. Any other reproduction or redistribution is strictly prohibited. All rights reserved.
This content is provided for test preparation purposes only and does not imply an endorsement by Mometrix of any particular political, scientific, or religious point of view.

Evaluation and Selection of Representative Images

Poststenotic Turbulence

Recall that the word "patent" refers to a structure that is open or clear. For example, a patent trachea (windpipe) is necessary for air to reach the lungs. When performing a carotid duplex exam, a patent artery is what the operator hopes to find. If a sonographer visualizes a stenosis on routine gray-scale imaging, a narrowing of the blood vessel lumen (opening) is present. If the user adds color Doppler, the direction of flow may vary as blood is attempting to enter and exit the stenotic region of the blood vessel. When pulsed-wave Doppler is used, the sonographer may expect to obtain higher flow velocities within the stenosis, but an even greater measurement distal to the stenosis. This is known as poststenotic turbulence, which is located after the blood vessel has been narrowed. Eddy currents will likely be visualized because the blood is no longer moving as smoothly as it was before the stenosis. If a clinician listens to the blood flow in this region, a bruit may be revealed.

Phasic, Pulsatile, and Steady Flow

Three types of blood flow that are witnessed in the circulatory systems of humans are phasic, pulsatile, and steady flow. Phasic flow is the typical flow pattern seen in veins. Phasic flow will exhibit velocity changes associated with breathing that causes red blood cells to speed up or slow down. Steady flow is constantly present in the venous system, and it takes place when the patient holds their breath. Steady flow does not vary in velocity; rather, it moves at the same speed. The heart is constantly contracting and relaxing, which will create velocities of blood flow that will fluctuate because of the movement of the heart wall, which is considered to be pulsatile. Pulsatile flow is also visualized in the arterial system because blood is moving at a greater velocity than it is in the venous system.

Doppler Principle

The method used to measure the velocity of blood flow within the body is called the Doppler principle. The frequency of sound varies as the distance between the transmitted frequency and receiver changes positions. If the distance between the sound source and receiver stays the same, the frequency will not be altered. An alteration of the frequency is called a Doppler shift or Doppler frequency. The Doppler shift is directly related to the velocity of blood within the circulatory system. Keep in mind that the velocity includes the speed (magnitude) and direction of blood flow. Slower velocities will cause a lower Doppler frequency. A higher velocity will create a greater Doppler shift. Blood flow velocities are reported with units of meters per second (m/s).

Mirror Imaging Artifacts

A mirror artifact will always be visualized at a depth greater than that of the actual structure being imaged. This is known as a mirror artifact because a very strong reflector tends to redirect the sound waves as it strikes the mirror. This mirror will appear between the actual object being imaged and the second copy of the structure. The second copy will be an equal distance from the reflector as the object, but, as discussed earlier, at a deeper depth. This artifact can appear not only in gray-scale imaging, but also during color Doppler interrogation. In this case, a second vessel may appear deeper than the actual vessel, but it is actually a mirror artifact. When imaging the abdomen, a common mirror imaging artifact visualized is lung tissue on either side of the diaphragm, which is seen as a bright reflector.

Copyright © Mometrix Media. You have been licensed one copy of this document for personal use only. Any other reproduction or redistribution is strictly prohibited. All rights reserved.
This content is provided for test preparation purposes only and does not imply an endorsement by Mometrix of any particular political, scientific, or religious point of view.

Enhancement Artifacts

While imaging a structure that is fluid filled, for example, a cyst or the gallbladder, the tissue that is visualized posterior to these structures often appears extremely echogenic. The artifact that is the opposite of shadowing is known as an enhancement artifact. These fluid-filled structures visualized are the result of a lower rate of attenuation than the tissue that surrounds it, so structures below them may appear brighter. Shadowing produces a hypoechoic area behind an object that is highly attenuating and can prohibit one's ability to see the structures that extend underneath these structures. Enhancement can be of diagnostic value because radiologists rely on this enhancement artifact to reassure them that a structure is cystic.

Shadowing Artifacts

Shadowing is visualized when a highly attenuating structure is situated just above this artifact. Shadowing artifacts can often prevent the user from seeing underlying anatomical structures, but they may also serve as a helpful diagnostic indicator during ultrasound exams. A shadowing artifact appears as a hypoechoic or anechoic area deep in the structure that is highly attenuating. Sonographers may notice shadowing posterior to calcifications such as kidney stones and gallstones to aid the radiologist in making a correct diagnosis. The artifact that appears completely different than those characteristics of a shadowing artifact is known as enhancement. In this case, a hyperechoic region appears deep to a structure that is weakly attenuating. Although the appearance of enhancement artifacts is very different, they provide the radiologist with helpful information when discerning tissues.

Refraction

Refraction is the bending of a sound beam when it travels from one medium to another. Two requirements must be met for refraction to take place in a clinical setting: (1) There must be an oblique incidence, and (2) the two media must be traveling at different speeds because refraction cannot take place if the media have identical speeds. Clinically, an ultrasound beam will only bend slightly at various tissue interfaces. Bone tends to create larger refraction angles because the speed of sound in bone is faster than the speed of sound in soft tissues. Snell's law is used to calculate refraction, and the following equation may be used:

$$\frac{\sin(\text{angle of transmission})}{\sin(\text{angle of incidence})} = \frac{\text{speed of medium 2}}{\text{speed of medium 1}}.$$

Reverberation Artifacts

Reverberation artifacts resemble a stepladder and will be in a location that is parallel to the ultrasound beam. Although the first two reflections closest to the probe actually exist, the numerous reflections deeper to them do not and are considered artifacts. These artifacts are created as an ultrasound signal bounces between two strong reflectors that are located parallel to the main axis of the ultrasound beam. These bright reflections resemble a stepladder because they contain several "rungs" and are evenly spaced. Another way to describe the appearance of a reverberation artifact is like a set of venetian blinds. These artifacts will always be the same distance from each other. If the distance is 0.5 cm between interfaces, the first reverberation will be 0.5 cm deeper than the object and will be seen at 1 cm. The next artifact will be at 1.5 cm, and the next will be at 2 until they can no longer be seen on the display.

Tissue Harmonics

Tissue harmonics are not contained within the ultrasound beam that is emitted from the transducer. Tissue harmonics are produced when the sound beam interacts with tissues that are deeper in the body in a nonlinear fashion. However, tissue harmonics do not occur when the

Copyright © Mometrix Media. You have been licensed one copy of this document for personal use only. Any other reproduction or redistribution is strictly prohibited. All rights reserved.
This content is provided for test preparation purposes only and does not imply an endorsement by Mometrix of any particular political, scientific, or religious point of view.

scanning depth is shallow. The sound beams that are transmitted must be strong; weak sound waves will not produce any tissue harmonics at all. Sound beams that are somewhat strong will only produce a small number of harmonics. With strong beams, the harmonics are created within the main line of the ultrasound wave. Tissue harmonics will only emerge from this main axis and will create very few imaging errors because of the strength of the beam.

Fundamental and Harmonic Frequencies

The fundamental frequency is the frequency of the ultrasound beam that is produced by the transducer and imparted into the patient. If a 6 MHz transducer is selected, 6 MHz will be the fundamental frequency. Harmonic imaging is a technology available to correct the malformation of the ultrasound wave that may take place when the fundamental frequency is used. If the sound beam is distorted, a diagnostic exam may not be possible. The harmonic frequency will be two times larger than the fundamental frequency. If the fundamental frequency is 6 MHz, the harmonic frequency is 12 MHz. An ultrasound beam that is created with harmonic frequencies will not undergo as much distortion and is less likely to produce images with artifact. When harmonics are used, a strong signal is required, and the signals will be located in the main axis of the sound wave.

Adjusting Color Scale to Correctly Display Color Flow

Aliasing can occur during pulsed-wave Doppler exams and when using color Doppler. Aliasing is visualized when the Doppler frequency is higher than what is known as the Nyquist limit. In this example, perhaps aliasing is visualized within an artery. The blood flow velocity within an artery is generally greater than the blood flow moving through a vein. The sonographer would need to raise the scale for color Doppler. This scale will be seen along the side of the image next to the color box. If the scale is increased, the aliasing should disappear, and the color box will display blood flow with only one color within the artery instead of many colors representing the artery. Keep in mind that an increase in the scale on the color Doppler function will not allow the system to pick up flow within veins because the velocity is lower.

Differentiating Between Flow Reversal and Aliasing

It is important for vascular technologists to realize that aliasing can occur not only with spectral Doppler analysis, but with color-flow Doppler as well. The user must be able to discern between aliasing and the reversal of flow (bidirectional flow). In order to determine if aliasing is present, the user must pay close attention to the color map located on the side of the image. If the colors on the map tend to wrap from the top around the outside and to the bottom of the map, then users may assume that aliasing is present. If the colors on the middle of the color map communicate with each other, then bidirectional flow is present. The best step an ultrasound user can take in order to remove an aliasing artifact from a color Doppler exam is to increase the level of the velocity scale.

Determining Direction of Blood Flow

While Using a Linear Probe When Steering Is Used

Vascular technologists should check the color map on the image to determine which colors represent the toward (above the baseline) and away (beneath the baseline) flow in a blood vessel. When the color box is angled, instead of a rectangle it is in the shape of a parallelogram. Users must find a landmark that can be thought of as the pretend location of the probe within the vessel. In order to do this, find the top corner of the steered color box and draw a line down. The imaginary line that does not bump into any other portion of the color box will be where the fictional probe is located. From the placement of the probe, determine if the color within the box is moving toward or away. The direction of blood flow is decided as you track either to or from the position of the transducer. This will either be a left-to-right or right-to-left movement.

Copyright © Mometrix Media. You have been licensed one copy of this document for personal use only. Any other reproduction or redistribution is strictly prohibited. All rights reserved.
This content is provided for test preparation purposes only and does not imply an endorsement by Mometrix of any particular political, scientific, or religious point of view.

Sector-Shaped Image with a Vessel That Is in a Horizontal Direction

Color flow in a sector-shaped image cannot be steered like it can with a linear transducer. Only the size and location can be adjusted. If a sector-shaped image contains a vessel that is in a horizontal direction, it is first important to find the color map to decide the color that represents flow moving toward the transducer (above the black line). The vascular technologist will notice that the color beneath the black line on the color map refers to blood moving away from the transducer. The user can then decide if the blood flow is moving from left to right (or right to left) by tracking it from the top color to the bottom color. This will make the direction of blood flow more apparent.

Importance of Doppler Angle When Measuring Velocities

In order for the vascular technologist to obtain the most accurate measurement during a carotid duplex exam, the moving red blood cells should be located parallel to the transducer. In this case, the measurement reflects the velocity located in all parts of the ultrasound wave. A positive Doppler frequency occurs when the velocity of the returning signals from blood cells moving toward the transducer is greater than the transmitted velocity. When the blood is not moving exactly parallel to the sound beam, the velocity that is measured will be a value that is not as accurate. For example, if the angle cursor is larger than the actual Doppler angle, the velocity will also be higher. If the angle cursor is lower than the angle that is parallel to the vessel wall, then the velocity will be underestimated.

Doppler Equation

When a vascular technologist is using gray scale during the ultrasound exam, the ideal incident beam is when the transducer is placed 90 degrees to the object being scanned. For Doppler, however, the maximum frequency shift will be obtained with an incident angle of either 0 degrees (blood flow moving toward the transducer) or 180 degrees (red blood cells moving away from the transducer). By using the Doppler equation, the cosine of 90 degrees is equal to 0, so we cannot measure any Doppler frequency when the incident beam is 90 degrees (perpendicular) to the direction of blood flow, so vascular technologists must be careful to not assume that the blood vessel is occluded because this is likely not the case. By changing the angle of the color box, the blood should be seen flowing once again.

Correlation of Blood Velocity to Spectral Broadening

Spectral analysis with pulsed-wave Doppler allows users to see, listen to, and measure various blood flow velocities. The spectral window is the clear black region between the baseline and the spectral line. When this area is filled in and there is widening of the line, spectral broadening is indicated. Spectral broadening is typical when turbulent (high-velocity) blood flow is sampled. This turbulence is comprised of many areas of flow reversal, and various velocities and flow may be seen beneath the baseline. If a carotid artery is being interrogated and the vascular technologist can visualize a tight stenosis, spectral broadening may be seen. It may also be present when small vessels are being investigated or if a sample is obtained at the point where a vessel bifurcates.

Aliasing

Aliasing is the phenomenon that takes place during a vascular ultrasound exam when the frequency exceeds half the PRF. When pulsed-wave Doppler is used, extremely high velocity blood flow can be difficult to measure accurately. When the blood flow looks as if it is moving in the wrong direction, this is known as aliasing. On spectral Doppler, this waveform will appear to wind around the baseline to look as if it is traveling in the wrong direction. The Nyquist limit is the most significant

Copyright © Mometrix Media. You have been licensed one copy of this document for personal use only. Any other reproduction or redistribution is strictly prohibited. All rights reserved.
This content is provided for test preparation purposes only and does not imply an endorsement by Mometrix of any particular political, scientific, or religious point of view.

velocity that can be accurately tracked before aliasing occurs. The formula that can be used to determine the Nyquist limit is

$$\text{Nyquist limit} = \frac{[\text{pulse repetition frequency (PRF)}]}{2}.$$

Aliasing can also take place when using color Doppler. If a slower PRF occurs because the color box is too wide or the depth is too great, aliasing may be visualized.

Copyright © Mometrix Media. You have been licensed one copy of this document for personal use only. Any other reproduction or redistribution is strictly prohibited. All rights reserved.
This content is provided for test preparation purposes only and does not imply an endorsement by Mometrix of any particular political, scientific, or religious point of view.

Procedures

Abdominal/Pelvic Vasculature

Aortoiliac Vasculature

Blood Flow from the Heart to the Abdominal Aorta

Oxygenated blood leaves the heart and is pumped into the aorta, which contains several arterial branches to carry the blood to all cells of the body. The aorta has four major sections and is the longest artery in the human body. From the left ventricle of the heart, the blood is first pumped into a short segment of the aorta known as the ascending aorta. Next, the oxygenated blood reaches the aortic arch before it becomes the descending (thoracic) aorta. The fourth segment arises once this blood vessel passes through a small opening in the diaphragm. Here, it is known as the abdominal aorta. It is the largest artery in the abdominal cavity, and it supplies the organs and tissues of the abdomen, pelvis, and lower extremities with oxygenated blood.

Blood Flow from the Distal Portion of the Abdominal Aorta

The thoracic aorta becomes the abdominal aorta once it passes through the diaphragm to carry oxygenated blood away from the heart. This artery eventually bifurcates at the level of the fourth lumbar vertebra to become the right and left common iliac arteries. These arteries extend to about the level of the last lumbar vertebra or proximal sacral region and eventually continue as the right and left external iliac arteries. These arteries descend to become the common femoral arteries as they descend inferior and laterally along the psoas muscle's medial margin. The external iliac arteries are referred as the right and left common femoral arteries once they have continued past (beneath) the right and left inguinal ligament. Conversely, the internal iliac (also referred to as the hypogastric) arteries actually branch off of and course medially to the common iliac arteries to supply oxygenated blood to the wall of the external genitalia, buttocks, thigh, and wall of the pelvis.

Innominate Artery

The ascending aorta becomes the aortic arch, which contains three major branches. The aortic arch is named as such because it curves up toward the back and then bends left prior to its plunge as the descending aorta. The first or most proximal branch that stems from the aortic arch is the innominate artery. This vessel is also known as the brachiocephalic artery or is even referenced as the brachiocephalic trunk of the aorta. This vessel is the branch that is the largest of the three branches of the aortic arch, and it supplies the right side of the brain, face, neck, and arm with

Copyright © Mometrix Media. You have been licensed one copy of this document for personal use only. Any other reproduction or redistribution is strictly prohibited. All rights reserved.
This content is provided for test preparation purposes only and does not imply an endorsement by Mometrix of any particular political, scientific, or religious point of view.

oxygenated blood. The innominate artery gives rise to the right CCA and the right subclavian artery. Notably, the innominate artery is only found on the right side of the body.

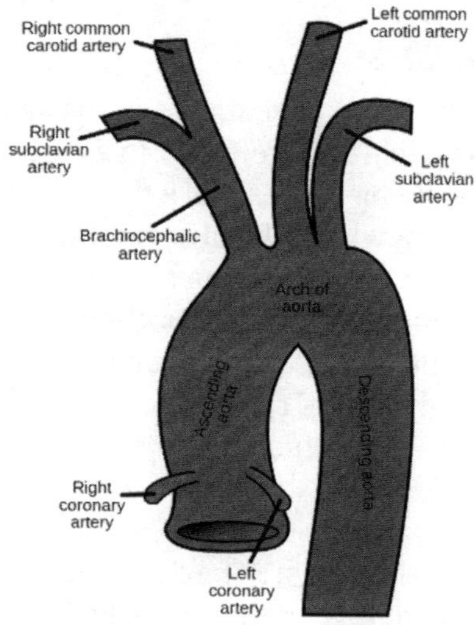

Anomalies Affecting the Aortic Arch

Anomalies of the aortic arch are called congenital malformations because they are present at birth. The first branch of the aorta is the innominate (also referred to as the brachiocephalic) artery. The second artery to stem from the aortic arch is the left common carotid artery (CCA), with the left subclavian artery as the third division. Although there are multiple anatomical arrangements outside of the normal configurations, the most common variation occurs when the innominate and left common carotid arteries arise from the same region of the aortic arch. Sometimes, the left CCA will originate from the innominate artery (however, this is a less common scenario). Another anomaly of the aortic arch is the visualization of the left vertebral artery that originates directly from the arch in a more proximal location than the left subclavian artery instead of branching from the left subclavian artery.

Complications Experienced by a Patient with a Known AAA

The aorta is the blood vessel that transports oxygenated blood from the left ventricle of the heart to all cells in the body. After the aorta passes through the diaphragm, it becomes the abdominal aorta, which bifurcates at the level of the fourth lumbar vertebra. Abdominal aortic aneurysms (AAAs) are frequently diagnosed sonographically, with nearly 30% being diagnosed as an incidental finding. Aneurysm rupture is a major complication. The probability of rupture increases when a patient is a smoker. Other complications include distal embolization, especially aneurysms seen in the extremities, but this could stem from the abdominal aorta as well. Individuals with an aneurysm are more prone to developing another aneurysm often in the popliteal or common femoral arteries. If a vascular technologist diagnoses a unilateral popliteal artery aneurysm, it may be beneficial to evaluate the contralateral popliteal artery because bilateral presence is not uncommon.

Size of the Aneurysm Warranting Surgical Repair

The aorta is the largest artery in the human body. After the aorta descends through the diaphragm, it becomes the abdominal aorta. The average diameter of the abdominal aorta in adults is approximately 2 cm narrowing slightly as it descends toward the aortic bifurcation. Women tend to have an aorta that is somewhat smaller than men, usually measuring 2–3 mm less. This is important to consider because an aorta that measures more than 3 cm is considered an AAA. Another characterization of an AAA is when the region is 1.5 times the diameter of the segment that is just

Copyright © Mometrix Media. You have been licensed one copy of this document for personal use only. Any other reproduction or redistribution is strictly prohibited. All rights reserved.
This content is provided for test preparation purposes only and does not imply an endorsement by Mometrix of any particular political, scientific, or religious point of view.

proximal in location. If the AAA has a measurement of 5.5 cm, then surgical repair is warranted because those that are larger than 6 cm have a 10%–20% risk of rupture. A 20%–40% chance of rupture accompanies an AAA that is 7 cm.

Fusiform vs. Saccular Aneurysms

An aneurysm is a dilation of an artery due to a weakness in the arterial wall that may develop in any artery. Abdominal aortic aneurysms, otherwise referred to as AAAs, materialize in the abdominal aorta and are diagnosed when the aorta measures more than 3 cm from outer wall to outer wall. Aneurysms are described to be fusiform when a focal segment of the blood vessel expands or bulges on all sides. Fusiform aneurysms tend to be the most common shape identified in aortic aneurysms, and they have ends that appear tapered. Another shape created by an aortic aneurysm is called a saccular aneurysm. This type often occurs when the patient has experienced trauma. The dilation is asymmetrical because it only occurs on one side of the vessel and tends to transpire in the thoracic aorta more often than the abdominal portion.

Measuring an Aneurysm

Ultrasound is the imaging modality of choice when performing abdominal aortic screenings for AAAs or as a follow-up method when an AAA was previously diagnosed with ultrasound or any other modality such as CT, MRI, or X-ray. An aneurysm is diagnosed when either a dilation of the artery is more than 3 cm or if a bulge seen has a diameter of 1.5 times more than a connecting segment of the aorta. Longitudinal and transverse images with AP measurements should be taken in the proximal, mid, and distal regions of the abdominal aorta. When an AAA is discovered during an ultrasound exam, the technologist should carefully document the location and size by measuring the aneurysm from outer wall to outer wall. In the transverse plane, the maximum diameter should be documented. It is not important to measure the length of the aneurysm, but it should be documented if the iliac arteries are also affected.

Aortic Dissection

An aortic dissection is a life-threatening condition that develops when there is a tear in the innermost layer of the arterial wall (referred to as the intima). This tear enables blood to seep into a false lumen, which is created between the inner and middle layers of the artery. When the true and false lumens are evaluated with color and spectral Doppler, they could demonstrate different directions and velocities. The false lumen will often demonstrate bidirectional, high-resistance flow, whereas normal spectral waveforms may be seen in the true lumen. Ultrasound findings will also display a hyperechoic flap or membrane that separates the true and false lumens. If the false lumen clots, no blood flow would be demonstrated with color Doppler. The thoracic aorta is the region in which dissections typically develop, but they can continue into the abdominal and even the iliac arteries. People that have Marfan syndrome are genetically predisposed to aortic dissections as are those that experience trauma.

Aortic Ectasia

Ectasia of the aorta is suspected when there is a general dilation of the artery that has not yet reached aneurysmal dimensions. A standard measurement of the abdominal aorta is 3 cm or less when measured from outer wall to outer wall or if the diameter is 1.5 times less than what the more proximal connecting segment of the abdominal aorta measures. Individuals that have been diagnosed with ectasia have a higher incidence of developing an aneurysm because this swelling may continue to evolve; follow-up ultrasounds are often performed to evaluate this progression. Ectasia of the aorta may be seen when interrogating the thoracic, abdominal, and even the common iliac arteries.

Copyright © Mometrix Media. You have been licensed one copy of this document for personal use only. Any other reproduction or redistribution is strictly prohibited. All rights reserved.
This content is provided for test preparation purposes only and does not imply an endorsement by Mometrix of any particular political, scientific, or religious point of view.

Using Extended Field of View Control

When the vascular technologist would like to visualize as much of the abdominal aorta as possible at one time, the extended field of view control on the ultrasound system should be used. This panoramic image is available on most modern ultrasound equipment, and it replaces the split-screen method of demonstrating objects that are longer than the transducer face. By acquiring various volume data, the system will stitch the information together in order to display one image. This single image will offer clinicians the ability to visualize the majority of the structure at the same time. This application can be used when interrogating the abdominal aorta, and it may provide additional information regarding the exact location of aneurysms or ectasia that may be encountered. Often, anatomical structures are enlarged and may be difficult to obtain measurements from.

Region of Abdominal Aorta with the Highest Incidence of Aneurysms

When a vascular technologist is evaluating the abdominal aorta, longitudinal and transverse images with measurements should be performed. Proximal images and measurements should be taken in the vicinity of the origin of the celiac artery below the diaphragm. The region in which the renal arteries start is where the measurements should be labeled as mid aorta. The distal region of the abdominal aorta is measured just prior to where the aorta bifurcates to become the right and left common iliac arteries. The majority of AAAs are found in the distal segment of the abdominal aorta and considered to be infrarenal in location. Infrarenal describes the area below the origin of the renal arteries.

Coarctation of the Aorta

Coarctation of the aorta is a congenital heart defect that develops because of a constriction of or the narrowing of the aorta. This narrowing often develops distal to the origin point of the left subclavian artery and may be found in conjunction with other heart conditions, but it can also affect the abdominal aorta. Depending on the severity of this narrowing of the aorta, the patient may be diagnosed at different ages and a mild case may not be diagnosed until the individual develops hypertension, whereas others are diagnosed with this condition shortly after birth. This narrowing can often be seen on gray-scale and color Doppler images. In children and young adults that have abnormal renal artery duplex studies in addition to high blood pressure, a coarctation of the aorta should be suspected.

Leriche Syndrome

Leriche syndrome is the result of an obstruction of the distal aorta that is typically found in males between the ages of 30 and 40. This is different from most cases of occlusive disease of the abdominal aorta because it is seen more often in older populations that have significant atherosclerosis. Acute and chronic cases have been diagnosed, with acute onset seen more often in females. Male patients with chronic cases of Leriche syndrome often present with the triad of decreased or absent femoral pulses; intermittent claudication of the pelvis, thighs, and calves; and erectile dysfunction. Still other symptoms include coldness of the lower extremities, pain, and numbness of the extremities. Over time, there is progression of the occlusion, which is typically proximal to the aortic bifurcation but may extend proximally and distally into the iliac and femoral arteries.

Takayasu's Arteritis

Takayasu's arteritis is a condition in which the walls of the aorta and its branches become thickened due to inflammation. This thickening of the arterial walls eventually leads to vessels that are stenotic and that may become occluded over time. One of the main symptoms of this disorder is

Copyright © Mometrix Media. You have been licensed one copy of this document for personal use only. Any other reproduction or redistribution is strictly prohibited. All rights reserved.
This content is provided for test preparation purposes only and does not imply an endorsement by Mometrix of any particular political, scientific, or religious point of view.

a reduced or even a complete inability to find a pulse in the patient's extremities. Other symptoms are dizziness, vertigo, headaches, and hypertension, and even heart attacks and strokes have been reported. This condition is rare and is typically seen in women that are younger than 40 (and in some cases even in their teenage years) and is believed to be an autoimmune disorder. The narrowed vessels may be seen in gray-scale ultrasound imaging, but angiography is the modality that is used most often to make an accurate diagnosis of Takayasu's arteritis.

Aortobifemoral Bypass Graft

A bypass graft acts as a conduit that gives blood a different route to avoid an occlusion or serious stenosis. The purpose of a lower extremity bypass graft is to carry oxygenated blood around the lesion(s) within the artery that is (are) obstructing blood flow. This conduit must connect the region of the artery above the stenosis or occlusion with a region that is located below the area of the stenosis or occlusion in order to reestablish blood flow to both legs, which requires patent vessels in the proximal and distal locations. An aortobifemoral bypass graft is necessary in a patient that suffers from significant iliac artery disease that affects the right and left iliac arteries.

Celiac Trunk and Its Branches

The celiac trunk (also referred to as the celiac axis) is found in the abdomen and supplies blood to various digestive organs. The celiac trunk originates from the anterior surface of the abdominal aorta as the first branch. The celiac trunk is a short segment that gives off three main branches, which are the splenic, left gastric, and common hepatic arteries. The splenic artery supplies blood to the spleen, stomach, and the pancreas. The left gastric artery supplies blood to the stomach and esophagus. The common hepatic artery supplies blood to the liver as well as the gallbladder.

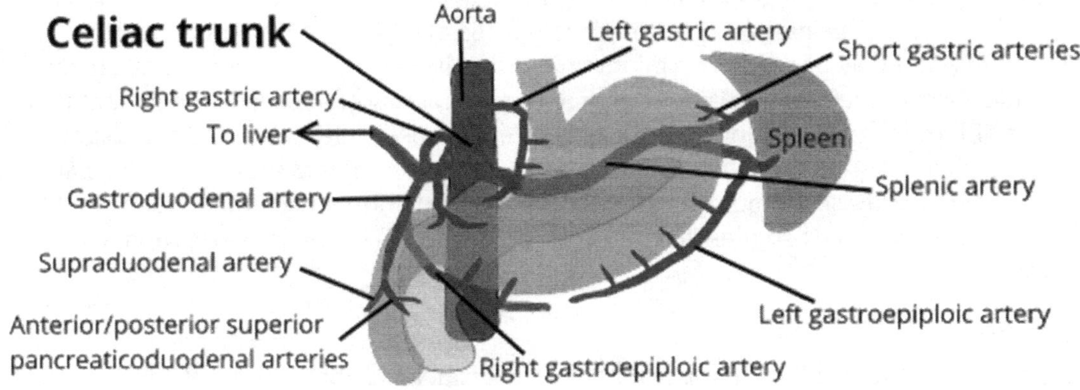

Examining the Celiac Artery with Ultrasound vs. CTA

Before starting an exam, vascular technologists are taught to always look at previous exams and/or imaging reports for comparison. Sometimes there can be a discrepancy in the findings, especially if a patient has undergone computed tomography angiography (CTA) to evaluate the mesenteric blood vessels. For example, if a patient presents with symptoms of median arcuate ligament syndrome, the CTA may appear normal because the exam is done while the patient suspends respiration upon deep inspiration. Even if the patient is positive for median arcuate ligament syndrome, the CTA may appear normal because often the deep breath can create this situation. Ultrasound, however, can be performed when the patient is in quiet respiration, deep inspiration, and even during expiration. The vascular technologist has the ability to scan the patient while lying on their back and also in an upright position. Having the patient sit or stand up causes the celiac artery to drop down into the abdomen more, which can alleviate the confinement on the celiac artery caused by the median arcuate ligament.

Copyright © Mometrix Media. You have been licensed one copy of this document for personal use only. Any other reproduction or redistribution is strictly prohibited. All rights reserved.
This content is provided for test preparation purposes only and does not imply an endorsement by Mometrix of any particular political, scientific, or religious point of view.

Celiac Artery Compression Syndrome

Celiac artery compression syndrome occurs when the median arcuate ligament travels anterior to the celiac artery (instead of above the point at which the celiac artery arises from the abdominal aorta), which can create severe pain when the artery is compressed by the ligament. This pain is often postprandial and may be accompanied by nausea, diarrhea, and weight loss. Physicians may also hear a bruit in the epigastric region that may fluctuate with the patient's breathing. The pain may be caused by the compression of the nerves in the area of the celiac artery, or it could be due to the decreased perfusion to the digestive organs. Ultrasound can be used to examine the celiac axis in multiple patient positions, fasting states, and with various breathing techniques to determine the cause. If the PSV is more than 200 cm/s in the fasting state, it is highly suspicious for a significant stenosis or occlusion of the celiac artery. Celiac artery compression syndrome is also referred to as median arcuate ligament syndrome.

Hepatic Arterial vs. Portal Blood Flow to the Liver

Blood reaches the liver from two pathways: the hepatic arterial system and the portal system. The hepatic artery is a branch of the celiac artery, which is the first branch of the abdominal aorta. Although the hepatic artery supplies the majority of the oxygenated blood that the liver receives, it is actually only responsible for transporting about 25%–30% of the total blood volume into the liver. The rest of the blood volume (70%–75%) is transported to the liver from the main portal vein. Most of the blood that the portal vein transports has been depleted of oxygen and is traveling from the intestines to the liver to be cleaned. Portal veins tend to have a bright wall in a normal liver, whereas the hepatic arteries do not have echogenic walls. After the blood circulates through the liver, it is returned to the IVC from the hepatic veins.

Rayleigh Scattering During an Exam

Scattering is an erratic, unsystematic diversion of the ultrasound beam in multiple directions. Rayleigh scattering is just one type of scattering, but instead of being erratic, the sound wave is directed in 360 degrees in an organized manner. Rayleigh scattering takes place because the actual size of the target is much smaller than the wavelength of the ultrasound beam. For example, if a vascular technologist can visualize blood flow in hepatic vessels without color-flow Doppler, it is due to Rayleigh scattering. The red blood cells are the target of the ultrasound system, but the image may be misinterpreted because without color flow the vessels may appear as if they are clotted. If the user decreases the frequency, then the signal amplitude of what may appear as a clot in the hepatic vessels should be less apparent. Rayleigh scattering is proportional to the frequency to the fourth power.

Placement of a TIPS

A transjugular intrahepatic portosystemic shunt (TIPS) is a low-resistance conduit that is created to establish a connection between the right branch of the portal vein and the hepatic vein. This procedure is performed under fluoroscopy by an interventional radiologist. The right jugular vein is the preferred access site to reach the hepatic vein because the liver is accessed from the superior and inferior vena cava. Once the catheter is within the hepatic vein, the pressure gradient in the liver is measured to help determine the extent of PHTN. TIPS is a highly successful therapeutic procedure for patients with cirrhosis who have developed PHTN or esophageal varices, and some individuals with ascites have had success with this kind of treatment.

Use of Angle Correction During Spectral Doppler

Many venous flow studies do not require angle correction because the peak-systolic velocities (PSVs) are not measured. However, when evaluating a patient that has a transjugular intrahepatic

Copyright © Mometrix Media. You have been licensed one copy of this document for personal use only. Any other reproduction or redistribution is strictly prohibited. All rights reserved.
This content is provided for test preparation purposes only and does not imply an endorsement by Mometrix of any particular political, scientific, or religious point of view.

portosystemic shunt (TIPS), it is imperative for the vascular technologist to use angle correction during the spectral Doppler portions of the exam because the PSVs must be measured. Protocols after a TIPS procedure include using color Doppler of the portal vein to check the direction of the blood flow and for signs of thrombus or occlusion. Spectral Doppler includes measuring PSVs in the segments of the portal vein that supplies blood to the TIPS, and the proximal, mid, and distal regions of the TIPS. It is also important to measure blood flow distal to the TIPS in the hepatic vein. These PSVs should be measured with angle correction in mind, and the angle should be equal to or less than 60 degrees.

Superior Mesenteric Artery

The second main artery to branch from the abdominal aorta is the superior mesenteric artery (SMA). The origin of the SMA is roughly 1 cm from the point at which the first branch of the abdominal aorta stems from. This arterial trunk is named the celiac axis. However, in some patients the celiac artery and SMA may emerge from the same trunk. The SMA branches off the abdominal aorta anteriorly and then runs posterior to the pancreatic neck and splenic vein. Several important branches of the SMA supply oxygenated blood to the digestive system, especially those on the right side of the body. The cecum (which is the first portion of the colon) and ascending colon are on the right side of the patient's body and converge with the right half of the transverse colon and are all fed by the branches of the SMA.

Perfusion of Normal Mesenteric Arteries

Vascular technologists should be aware that blood flow in the SMA is vastly different in fasting and postprandial states. When the patient has been fasting, the SMA should display a high-resistance waveform with flow reversal. The postprandial spectral Doppler waveform should demonstrate more blood flow in order to aid in digestion and will therefore have a higher peak-systolic velocity (PSV) and end-diastolic velocity (EDV). This increase in flow is the result of the vasodilation of arteries that supply oxygenated blood to the organs of digestion. The waveform of the celiac artery will not be altered when scanned after the patient eats. Some protocols include having the patient drink a high-caloric drink especially if he or she has a mesenteric bypass graft to compare the blood flow before and after eating.

Celiac, Superior Mesenteric, and Inferior Mesenteric Arteries

The organs of digestion are fed by three main vessels: the celiac artery, the superior mesenteric artery (SMA), and the inferior mesenteric artery. In a patient presenting with intestinal ischemia, two out of the three blood vessels must demonstrate a significant stenosis with the SMA acting as the artery that supplies the majority of oxygenated blood to the intestines. Vascular technologists will not encounter chronic mesenteric ischemia very often, but when it is present, it develops from atherosclerotic disease. Another reason that chronic mesenteric ischemia is rare is because of the collateral channels that enable the blood to flow to the digestive organs. The arc of Riolan and gastroduodenal artery are two such vessels that keep blood flowing in the presence of a significant stenosis.

Symptoms of Diseased Mesenteric Arteries

Patients that have chronic mesenteric ischemia may experience nausea, vomiting, and diarrhea. Patients may experience weight loss because of the pain that is experienced when they eat, so they often avoid food. Postprandial pain is a common symptom of bowel ischemia, and it occurs after meals when there is more of a need for blood to reach the intestines. This is also known as bowel claudication because the symptoms arise after there is a need for an increased supply of blood or intestinal ischemia. An abdominal bruit may be present as well. Females are often at a higher risk of suffering from acute mesenteric ischemia, especially those women that are within the age group of

Copyright © Mometrix Media. You have been licensed one copy of this document for personal use only. Any other reproduction or redistribution is strictly prohibited. All rights reserved.
This content is provided for test preparation purposes only and does not imply an endorsement by Mometrix of any particular political, scientific, or religious point of view.

60 to 80 years old. Most cases of chronic mesenteric ischemia are due to significant stenosis of the SMA as well as either the celiac or inferior mesenteric artery.

Calculating the Resistive Index

Calculate the resistive index (RI) if the PSV of an arcuate renal artery is 41 cm/s and the EDV is 12 cm/s.

The resistive index (RI) is calculated during certain exams to measure how pulsatile blood flow is due to the peripheral resistance that is found in a more distal location than where the blood flow is being measured. The RI is calculated with the following formula: $\mathrm{RI} = \frac{\mathrm{PSV-EDV}}{\mathrm{PSV}}$. By plugging the known values into the formula, we can calculate the RI as follows: $\frac{41-12}{41} = \frac{29}{41} = 0.71$.

If the RI is calculated during a renal arterial duplex, it is considered abnormal if the RI is greater than or equal to 0.7, and normal if the value is less than 0.7.

Challenges in Identifying the Renal Arteries

Visualization of the renal arteries is often technically challenging due to bowel gas that can obstruct the image. The patient should fast prior to this exam to decrease the amount of bowel gas that will obscure the renal arteries. The vascular technologist should use a 3–5 MHz curvilinear transducer to help penetrate the patient's abdomen. The origin of the renal arteries is slightly distal to where the SMA branches from the abdominal aorta. Many vascular labs require the kidneys as well as the abdominal aorta to be examined as part of a renal artery Doppler exam. If the origins of the renal arteries are not well visualized from the anterior approach, it may be useful to turn the patient on his or her left side to use a coronal approach for what is known as the "banana peel" sign to locate the origins of the right and left renal arteries. Color Doppler is recommended to help the technologist locate these vessels.

Blood Flow from the Renal Hilum to the Renal Cortex

The renal arteries supply oxygenated blood traveling from the abdominal aorta to the adrenal glands, ureters, as well as the kidneys. Once the main renal artery enters the renal hilum, it branches into five segmental arteries that supply the various regions of the kidney. As these vessels travel further outward to the periphery of the kidney, they branch to become the interlobar arteries. These arteries are found near the renal pyramids. The arcuate arteries tend to curve around the base of the renal pyramids to finally supply blood to the renal cortex. These arteries are known as the interlobular arteries. Blood flow from the renal hilum to the cortex is as follows:

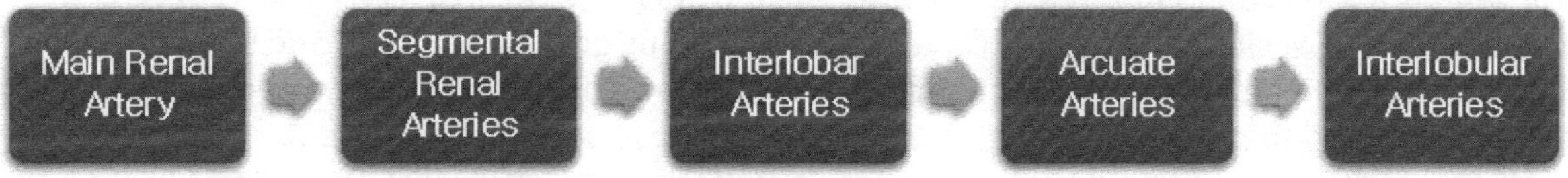

Main Renal Artery → Segmental Renal Arteries → Interlobar Arteries → Arcuate Arteries → Interlobular Arteries

Performing a Renal Arterial Duplex Exam

Many labs require the vascular technologist to image the abdominal aorta as well as the kidneys to assess the size and to look for any pathology that may be present. Typically, the blood flow in the renal arteries is seen as being of low resistance, while the aortic flow is of high resistance. In the proximal, mid, and distal segments of the renal arteries, the peak systolic and end-diastolic velocities are measured bilaterally. The peak systolic and end-diastolic velocities should also be sampled in the upper and lower poles within the segmental arteries and possibly the interlobar arteries. The renal-to-aortic ratio is calculated, and normal values will fall below 3.5. If the renal-to-

Copyright © Mometrix Media. You have been licensed one copy of this document for personal use only. Any other reproduction or redistribution is strictly prohibited. All rights reserved.
This content is provided for test preparation purposes only and does not imply an endorsement by Mometrix of any particular political, scientific, or religious point of view.

aortic ratio is greater than or equal to 3.5, this suggests that a significant stenosis is present. The renal-to-aortic ratio is calculated by dividing the greatest peak-systolic velocity (PSV) of the renal artery by the greatest PSV of the abdominal aorta.

Typical Visualization of Atherosclerosis

Renal artery stenosis can stem from many conditions including atherosclerosis and thrombosis, embolism, and fibromuscular dysplasia. When a renal artery duplex exam is performed, the kidneys and abdominal aorta are also interrogated. When atherosclerosis is present in the renal arteries, it tends to be present in the proximal segment of the renal arteries where they branch from the abdominal aorta. If the mid and distal segments are diseased, it tends to be the result of fibromuscular dysplasia. Proximal renal artery stenosis can be assumed when the renal/aortic velocity ratio has been calculated as being greater than 3.5.

Common Congenital Anomaly of the Renal Artery

The renal arteries originate from the abdominal aorta and carry oxygenated blood to the kidneys. Typically, most patients have two kidneys (one on either side of the spine). These organs are supplied by the renal artery, and although most individuals only have one renal artery on each side, it is not uncommon to see more than one renal artery. In fact, the most common congenital anomaly of the renal artery is multiple arteries that supply the kidneys, which is seen in roughly 30% of people. This can occur unilaterally, and when it is unilateral, it seems to develop on either side with equal prevalence but can also be found bilaterally in the same patient. Just like patients that only have one renal artery per side, multiple arteries typically stem from the same region of the aorta in those patients. However, they may also arise from the superior or inferior mesenteric arteries or even the common iliacs. In patients with congenital variants of the urinary system such as horseshoe or ectopic kidneys, it is not uncommon to see variations where the renal arteries arise.

Renal Artery with Reversal of Flow During Diastole

The renal arteries have low-resistance flow because these blood vessels are carrying blood to the kidneys, which are extremely vascular organs. Spectral analysis will demonstrate an arterial waveform of high resistance if the patient has kidney disease. A normal renal artery should also have an acceleration index of greater than 300 cm/s^2. If the waveform of the renal artery has a reversal of flow during diastole (which is not normal), the vascular technologist must carefully evaluate the ipsilateral renal vein. If there is a thrombus present in the renal vein, it could create outflow obstruction, which could cause the reversal of flow in diastole of the renal artery.

Renal/Aortic Ratio

Ultrasound is a useful and noninvasive modality to help diagnose renal artery stenosis. It is important to use a system that has the capability of providing gray-scale, color, and spectral Doppler functions to make sure that the correct vessel is being interrogated. One of the calculations that the ultrasound machine can provide is the renal/aortic ratio, which is a comparison of the highest PSV of the main renal artery to the aortic PSV. If the computed value of the systolic renal/aortic velocity is greater than 3.5, this suggests the possibility of a renal artery stenosis of 60% or more.

Blood Flow from the External Iliac Artery

Recall that the arterial system carries oxygenated blood from the heart. As the blood flows away from the heart and into the abdominal aorta bifurcation, it is directed toward the right and left common iliac arteries at the level of the fourth lumbar vertebra. This bifurcation enables these vessels to carry blood to the pelvis via the internal iliac (hypogastric) artery and lower extremities via the external iliac arteries. The external iliac artery is the result of another bifurcation of the

Copyright © Mometrix Media. You have been licensed one copy of this document for personal use only. Any other reproduction or redistribution is strictly prohibited. All rights reserved.
This content is provided for test preparation purposes only and does not imply an endorsement by Mometrix of any particular political, scientific, or religious point of view.

common iliac artery as it branches into the internal and external iliac arteries. The external iliac artery continues down the leg to become the common femoral artery (CFA) once it travels under the inguinal ligament. The CFA continues down the thigh and becomes the femoral artery to eventually become the popliteal artery once it reaches the posterior region of the knee.

Signal Found in the CFA If Significant Aortoiliac Lesion

It is essential to correctly diagnose patients that have aortoiliac lesions to aid in the treatment of peripheral arterial disease (PAD). In some cases, the distal region of the aorta and the proximal portion of the common iliac arteries are difficult to evaluate well due to bowel gas and the depth of these structures. Evaluation of the common femoral artery (CFA) may be useful when Doppler evaluation of the aortoiliac region is not possible. Spectral Doppler of a normal CFA will demonstrate a waveform that is triphasic with a reversal of flow seen below the baseline with a clean spectral window. In patients that present with a significant aortoiliac lesion, the CFA waveform will appear monophasic. If there is a total proximal occlusion, then collaterals feed the extremities and demonstrate a dampened signal as long as the occlusion was not acute.

Waveform That Demonstrates Tardus Parvus

Tardus parvus is a term that is used to describe how a pulse-wave spectral Doppler waveform appears when there is a more proximal stenosis present. Characteristics of a tardus parvus waveform include a delayed acceleration (which is also often referred to as a slow upstroke). The waveform will also have a more rounded (dampened) peak systolic appearance. This pattern could be seen in the left common iliac artery if there is an obstruction of the abdominal aorta. This pattern is also commonly seen when there is significant proximal stenosis of any artery in the body. Tardus parvus is commonly seen distal to a stenosis in the renal artery or if collateral channels have formed in the case of a total arterial occlusion.

Determining Thrombus in the IVC Using Ultrasound

Ultrasound is a cost-effective and noninvasive tool that can be used to quickly diagnose medical emergencies. Ultrasound can be performed bedside so that the patient does not have to be taken to the radiology department. The inferior vena cava (IVC) is located to the right of the abdominal aorta, and it returns blood from the lower body to the right atrium of the heart. The IVC is formed when the right and left common iliac veins join within the retroperitoneum. A thrombus (blood clot) may be readily identified in the IVC because it appears as an echogenic filling defect within the lumen of the IVC; a blood clot within the IVC is life-threatening. Color Doppler can also be used to demonstrate the incomplete saturation of color within the vessel. A thrombus in the IVC is typically the result of a deep vein thrombosis of the legs. An IVC filter may be placed in patients that cannot take anticoagulants to prevent emboli from lodging within the lungs or heart.

Position of the Left Renal Vein and the Abdominal Aorta

The right and left renal veins carry deoxygenated blood away from the kidneys into the IVC to be returned to the heart. The IVC is situated to the right of the midline in the abdomen, so the left renal vein must travel a greater distance than the right renal vein to return the blood into the IVC. The abdominal aorta is just to the left of the midline, which means that the left renal vein must cross anterior to the abdominal aorta before reaching the IVC. In a transverse plane, the left renal vein is seen between the SMA and the abdominal aorta, which may be another way to locate the left renal artery during a Doppler exam because it is anterior to the left renal artery.

Inferior Vena Cava and the Abdominal Aorta

The inferior vena cava (IVC) is a large vein that returns blood that has been depleted of oxygen back to the right atrium of the heart. The blood that is emptied into the IVC is from the level below the

Copyright © Mometrix Media. You have been licensed one copy of this document for personal use only. Any other reproduction or redistribution is strictly prohibited. All rights reserved.
This content is provided for test preparation purposes only and does not imply an endorsement by Mometrix of any particular political, scientific, or religious point of view.

heart. The IVC sits to the right of the spine and is formed by the confluence of the common iliac veins. This confluence is usually found at the level of the fifth lumbar vertebra. The abdominal aorta carries oxygenated blood and is a continuance of the thoracic aorta once it passes through the diaphragm and sits to the left side of the spine. At the level of the fourth lumbar vertebra, the abdominal aorta bifurcates into the right and left common iliac arteries, which continue down each lower extremity. The distal portion of the abdominal aorta tends to sit anterior to the IVC; therefore, the right common iliac arteries are found in front of the common iliac veins. The aortic bifurcation is proximal to the location in which the common iliac veins merge to form the IVC.

Budd-Chiari Syndrome

The blood within the liver is returned to the IVC via the right, middle, and left hepatic veins. Budd-Chiari syndrome is a condition in which thrombus is present within the hepatic veins. If these vessels are clotted, then the blood within the liver cannot be returned to the heart, which can lead to further problems such as PHTN. Gray-scale imaging will demonstrate filling defects within the hepatic vein(s). Collateral channels may be visualized along with splenomegaly and ascites. Color and spectral Doppler should be used as well to prove the absence of flow within these vessels. The patient's liver function tests will likely be higher than normal, and the patient may experience abdominal pain. Budd-Chiari syndrome may stem from tumor invasion or thrombus within the IVC, so it is important to carefully examine this structure.

Hepatofugal Blood Flow

The liver is one of the most vascular organs that humans have because of its dual blood supply. Not only does the hepatic artery carry oxygenated blood to the liver, but the portal venous system also transports blood into the liver from the digestive system. Hepatofugal flow is an abnormality of the direction of blood flow that takes place when flow patterns within the venous portal system move away from the liver instead of toward the liver. This occurs most commonly because of the pressure buildup in the portal system such as in the case of patients with cirrhosis, which will often result in PHTN. The diagnosis of hepatofugal flow is important to discern because it is often linked to a reduced survival outcome in patients with cirrhosis or patients that have had a liver transplant. The hepatic veins also demonstrate hepatofugal flow as they carry blood away from the liver and dump it into the IVC.

Using Shallow Breathing in the Ultrasound Study

When the IVC is of interest, it should be evaluated with gray-scale, color, and pulsed-wave Doppler by using a curvilinear transducer. An exhaustive scan of the liver should also be completed in addition to the hepatic veins. The hepatic veins return blood from the liver into the IVC. If a blood clot is present within the IVC, it should be seen with gray-scale imaging. In addition, the ultrasound user should also evaluate with color and spectral Doppler because these methods can provide additional information within the blood vessel as well as gather waveforms. The IVC and hepatic veins should be studied when the patient is breathing normally because deep breaths will compress the IVC and cause the forward flow to stop momentarily. The normal waveform of the IVC should demonstrate pulsatility due to the close proximity to the heart. If this pulsatility is absent or the waveform appears dampened, then a central IVC obstruction is possible.

Scenario

While using gray-scale ultrasound, a blood clot is visualized in the IVC. Explain why this clot will reach the right atrium prior to any other chamber of the heart.

Arteries are the vessels that carry oxygenated blood to all cells in the body. Once the cells have taken from the blood the nutrients and oxygen that they need, the blood is returned to the right side

Copyright © Mometrix Media. You have been licensed one copy of this document for personal use only. Any other reproduction or redistribution is strictly prohibited. All rights reserved.
This content is provided for test preparation purposes only and does not imply an endorsement by Mometrix of any particular political, scientific, or religious point of view.

of the heart before reaching the lungs to pick up oxygen once again. Blood that has been depleted of oxygen from the level above the heart is emptied into the SVC, which dumps blood into the right atrium of the heart. Blood is returned from the level below the heart from the IVC, which also empties into the right atrium. If a clot is present in the IVC and it breaks off, it will first travel to the right atrium, which is the first of the four chambers of the heart that blood travels in.

Use of an IVC Filter

An IVC filter is a device that is used for patients diagnosed with DVT of the veins within the pelvis or lower legs. Candidates for IVC filters have a history of blood clots but are unable to undergo anticoagulation therapy (blood thinners). These individuals are at an especially high risk of developing a PE, in which a blood clot breaks off and moves toward the heart and blocks the pulmonary artery, which could be fatal for the patient. Initially, IVC interruption devices were considered permanent devices, but today these medical devices can be removed if necessary or can even be put in place as a temporary solution for individuals having a surgery that puts them at a higher risk of developing a blood clot.

Placement of an IVC Filter

The IVC filter is a medical device that is used to capture and trap any blood clots that may have traveled from the pelvis or lower extremities to prevent them from reaching the heart and/or lungs. There are several vendors that manufacture vena cava interruption devices, and they are produced in various shapes (often shaped like a cone) and sizes, but they are metal filters that are inserted into the IVC at a level that is located slightly below the point at which the renal veins enter this structure. IVC filters are placed by either interventional radiologists or vascular surgeons by inserting a catheter (which contains a flat IVC filter) into the patient's groin or neck, which is fed into the IVC. Once the catheter is extracted, the filter remains in place and will open up to become fixated to the IVC vessel wall.

Portal and Hepatic Veins

The portal vein drains blood from the digestive system (including the associated glands). The union of the splenic and superior mesenteric veins forms the portal vein.

It divides into the left portal vein and the right portal vein before entering the liver. The left portal vein is smaller and located towards the front and top of the liver. The right portal vein is larger and located towards the back and bottom of the liver.

The hepatic veins are all of the veins that carry the blood from the liver. These veins terminate into three large veins (the right hepatic vein, the middle hepatic vein, and the left hepatic vein) that open into the inferior vena cava (IVC). The right hepatic vein is the largest and joins the IVC at the right side. The middle hepatic vein joins the IVC towards the front. The left hepatic vein is the smallest and joins the IVC towards the front.

Examining the Hepatic Veins During

Three hepatic veins are present within the liver; these are the right, middle, and left hepatic veins. These blood vessels remove deoxygenated blood from the liver by emptying the blood into the IVC to be returned to the right atrium of the heart. If the blood within the liver cannot be properly routed to the IVC, congestion of the liver can take place. This surplus of blood can impede liver function and cause PHTN. During a scenario such as this, PHTN is the result of a rise in pressure of the portal system when the hepatic veins are clotted. Tumor invasion can also be the cause of PTHN, so it is important to examine as much of the IVC in addition to the hepatic veins during an abdominal ultrasound.

Copyright © Mometrix Media. You have been licensed one copy of this document for personal use only. Any other reproduction or redistribution is strictly prohibited. All rights reserved.
This content is provided for test preparation purposes only and does not imply an endorsement by Mometrix of any particular political, scientific, or religious point of view.

Portal Vein and Its Branches

The main portal vein materializes from the confluence of several important vessels. These blood vessels drain the spleen and the intestines to transport blood to the liver in order to clear the blood of toxic materials. The splenic vein originates at the splenic hilum and passes posterior to the pancreatic tail and body until it reaches the head of the pancreas. Before the splenic vein reaches the head of the pancreas, it is joined by the inferior mesenteric vein. The landmark of the portal splenic confluence is found at the head of the pancreas where the splenic vein joins with the superior mesenteric vein. At the porta hepatis, this confluence emerges as the main portal vein, which divides into the left and right portal veins after it enters the liver. The left portal vein further divides into the lateral and medial branches within the left lobe of the liver. Once it reaches the right lobe of the liver, the right portal vein branches into anterior and posterior divisions.

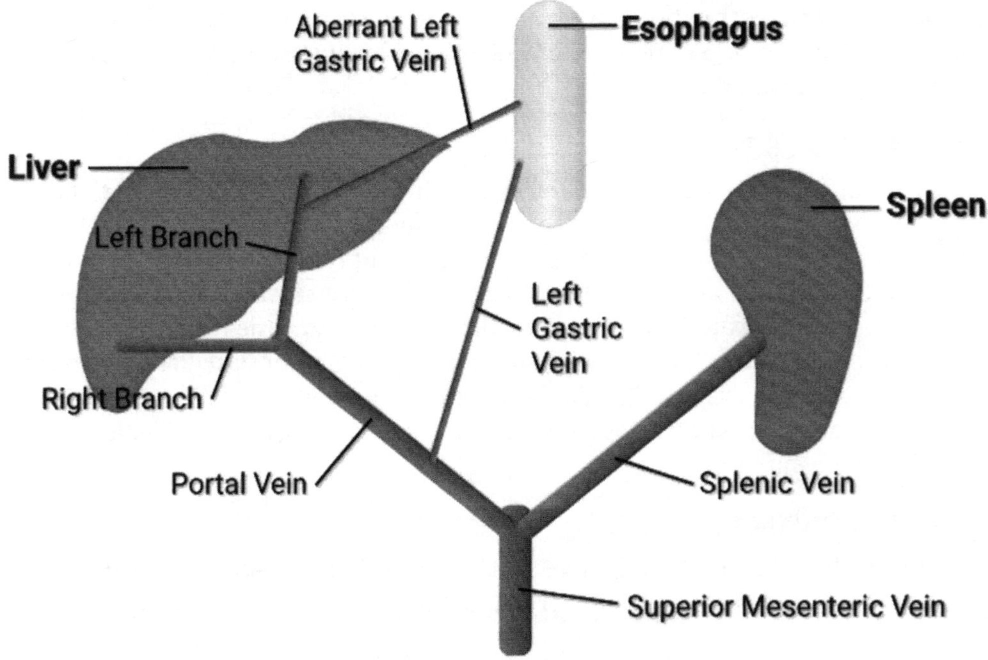

Hepatopetal Blood Flow

The portal veins carry blood from the intestines into the liver in order to remove any toxic substances before it is returned to the heart. Normal flow in the portal veins will demonstrate hepatopetal flow, which means that the flow is moving toward the liver. If the blood flow is traveling away from the liver, it is known as hepatofugal flow. There are several reasons that a patient may experience reduced hepatopetal flow, and some of the main causes are portal hypertension (PHTN), cirrhosis, a blood clot, or tumor formation as seen in hepatocellular carcinoma. Typically, the blood flow within the portal vein may be somewhat pulsatile, but it is continuous with small respiratory variations as the patient breathes in and out (phasicity).

Portal Hypertension

The liver is an essential organ: One of its functions is to eliminate toxins from the body. The portal vein transports a large percentage of blood from the bowel to the liver. When the pressure inside the portal system is elevated more than 5 mmHg than the pressure within the IVC, it is referred to as portal hypertension (PHTN). PHTN can be caused by several factors, such as anatomical variations that can lead to an increase of pressure or liver disease. Elevated pressures may be due to obstruction of the portal venous system or hepatic veins. Cirrhosis is often responsible for an

Copyright © Mometrix Media. You have been licensed one copy of this document for personal use only. Any other reproduction or redistribution is strictly prohibited. All rights reserved.
This content is provided for test preparation purposes only and does not imply an endorsement by Mometrix of any particular political, scientific, or religious point of view.

increase in resistance because scarring of the liver tissue reduces blood flow to the liver and increases pressure within the venous portal system.

Sonographic Findings Suggesting PHTN

There are many conditions that cause PHTN such as cirrhosis, pancreatitis, blood clots, and cancer. When scanning the liver, vascular technologists will typically notice portosystemic venous collaterals on gray-scale and color Doppler images. The portal vein may appear enlarged with a diameter of at least 13 mm, or it may demonstrate portal vein thrombosis, splenomegaly, or ascites. Pulsed-wave and color Doppler may demonstrate hepatofugal flow, which means that the blood is traveling in the wrong direction and away from the liver instead of the normal hepatopetal flow that moves toward the liver from the bowel. Clinically, the patient may present with gastrointestinal bleeding and leg edema, and dilated veins may be visualized on the abdominal wall of the patient.

Life-Threatening Esophageal Varices

When the submucosal veins of the inferior portion of the esophagus become distended, it indicates that esophageal varices are present. This is a serious complication of PHTN because bleeding can occur, and if it isn't diagnosed and managed quickly, a significant amount of bleeding can occur. If these vessels rupture, it can be deadly for the patient. In those with PHTN, the blood flowing into the liver is reduced. The coronary (gastric) vein will typically carry blood into the splenic vein (which joins the superior mesenteric vein to form the main portal vein). The veins that tend to empty into the portal system can no longer continue this function, so they end up dumping into the other vessels known as collateral channels. This rise in pressure causes the coronary vein blood to flow in the other direction, which creates esophageal varices.

Dilated Coronary Vein's Role in PHTN

Veins in the upper two-thirds of the esophagus return deoxygenated blood into the azygos vein, which eventually carries blood to the right atrium via the superior vena cava. These vessels do not play a role in the evolution of the dilated submucosal veins that are found in the inferior third portion of the esophagus known as esophageal varices. The coronary vein (also referred to as the left gastric vein) is a small vessel that has a diameter of about 1 mm. When this vein becomes dilated due to PHTN, it can reach a diameter of 1–2 cm, which can cause severe bleeding and even death. The coronary vein transports blood to the portal vein, but if PHTN is present, the direction of blood flow may reverse and end up emptying into the collateral varices instead.

Purpose and Length of the Renal Veins

The purpose of the renal veins is to carry blood that has been depleted of oxygen back to the heart. These vessels drain into the IVC so that the blood can be returned to the right atrium. Recall that the IVC is situated to the right of the body, so the left renal vein is longer because it must extend across the midline of the body in order to reach the IVC. In fact, the left renal vein crosses in front of the abdominal aorta but underneath one of the anterior branches of the abdominal aorta known as the SMA. The right renal vein tends to be shorter because the IVC is already just to the right of midline, so it is a much shorter distance to the IVC.

Nutcracker Syndrome

Nutcracker syndrome may include two variations, both of which compress the left renal vein. The left renal vein originates at the renal hilum and must cross the midline of the body to empty into the IVC, which lies to the right of the spine. On the way to the IVC, the left renal vein passes in between the SMA and the abdominal aorta. When the blood within the left renal vein cannot flow normally because it is impeded by the SMA and/or the abdominal aorta, it becomes disrupted. If the left renal

Copyright © Mometrix Media. You have been licensed one copy of this document for personal use only. Any other reproduction or redistribution is strictly prohibited. All rights reserved.
This content is provided for test preparation purposes only and does not imply an endorsement by Mometrix of any particular political, scientific, or religious point of view.

vein passes posterior to the abdominal aorta (referred to as the retroaortic left renal vein), it can also become compressed by the larger aorta, which can cause venous stasis.

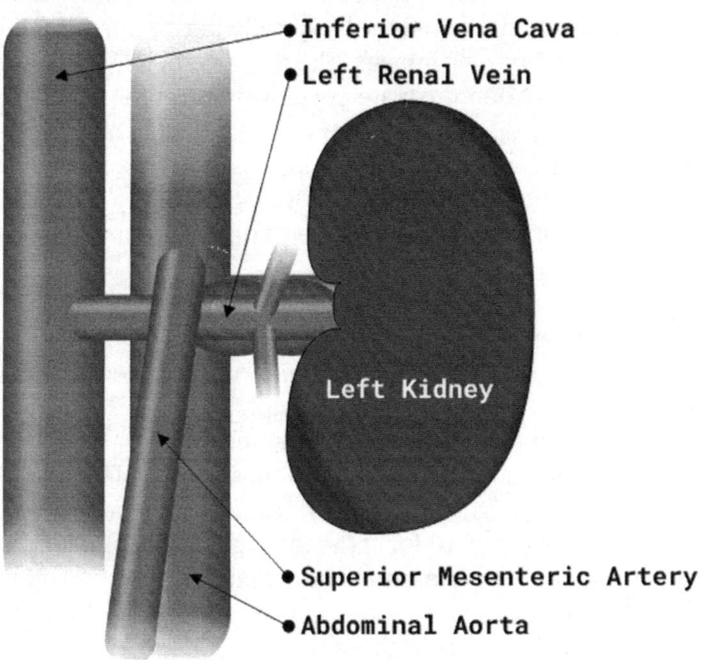

Evaluating the Renal Veins

The renal veins are responsible for returning blood that has been depleted of oxygen from the kidneys back to the heart. Typically, there is one renal vein for each kidney, but the ultrasound technologist may see more than one vessel on the same side. Renal veins empty the blood into the IVC so it can travel to the right atrium of the heart. The renal vein may develop a thrombus, especially if a clot is present in the IVC. Another condition of the renal veins that may be picked up during an ultrasound exam is a tumor invasion from a primary renal cell carcinoma. Vascular technologists should also evaluate the renal veins for possible compression of the left renal vein from the aorta or SMA as it travels between these two structures on the way to the IVC.

Major Veins in the Groin and Pelvis

The CFVs are found in the proximal portions of the thighs in the right and left lower extremities. As this vessel ascends into the groin, it becomes the external iliac vein at a level superior to the inguinal ligament. The common iliac vein is the result of the confluence of the internal iliac vein and the external iliac vein. The inferior vena cava (IVC) is the result of the right and left common iliac veins merging together in the abdomen typically at the level of the fifth lumbar vertebra. The IVC ascends in the abdomen just to the right of midline where it returns blood that has been depleted of oxygen to the right atrium of the heart.

Paraumbilical Vein

The paraumbilical vein starts at the umbilicus and travels between the layers of the falciform ligament and continues into the left portal vein. When visualized sonographically, it will have an anechoic and tubular configuration connecting the umbilicus to the falciform ligament. This blood vessel is important during pregnancy because it facilitates the transportation of oxygenated blood

Copyright © Mometrix Media. You have been licensed one copy of this document for personal use only. Any other reproduction or redistribution is strictly prohibited. All rights reserved.
This content is provided for test preparation purposes only and does not imply an endorsement by Mometrix of any particular political, scientific, or religious point of view.

from the placenta and carries it to the liver of the developing fetus via the umbilical cord. Ultrasound imaging of the paraumbilical vein is not usually possible because this blood vessel is not usually evident with sonography, even in the pediatric population. However, this blood vessel may become enlarged in individuals that have PHTN so that the pressure within the portal veins can be reduced when these channels recanalize so the blood in the paraumbilical vein can move the blood into the superficial epigastric vein. This vessel may recanalize in patients that have cirrhosis as well.

Pre/Post Surgical Ultrasound Examination for Liver Transplant

Ultrasound is a very useful tool in the pre and post operative evaluation of the liver patient. Prior to surgery ultrasound is used to evaluate:

- The health of liver tissue (hepatocytes).
- Identify lesions.
- Determine the openness and size of the portal vein, hepatic veins, and the inferior vena cava (IVC).
- Assess the biliary system for dialation.

After surgery, blood clot formation in the hepatic artery (thrombosis) is the most dangerous complication. Ultrasound is used to monitor the health of the hepatic vascular structures after surgery.

Thrombosis of the hepatic artery or portal vein may lead to massive death of liver cells (hepatic necrosis). The presence of air in the hepatic parenchyma (functional cells of the liver) shows up as shadowing on the sonogram. Gangrene of the liver is also apparent in the hepatic texture.

Some other things to monitor for are portal vein thrombosis and any blockages of the IVC and hepatic veins.

Anatomy of the Liver

The liver is the largest solid organ of the body. It is also the largest gland. It weighs about three pounds in an adult and is located below the diaphragm on the right side of the abdomen. The liver is made up of four **lobes**: right, left, quadrate, and caudate lobes. The liver is secured to the diaphragm and abdominal walls by five **ligaments**. They are called the falciform (which forms a membrane-like barrier between the right and left lobes), coronary, right triangular, left triangular, and round ligaments.

The liver processes blood once it has received nutrients from the intestines via the **hepatic portal vein**. The **hepatic artery** supplies oxygen-rich blood from the abdominal aorta so that the organ can function. Blood leaves the liver through the **hepatic veins**. The liver's functional units are called **lobules** (made up of layers of liver cells). Blood enters the lobules through branches of the portal vein and hepatic artery. The blood then flows through small channels called **sinusoids**.

Fissures of the Liver

The main lobar fissure definitively divides the liver into the right and left lobes. It is located along a line connecting the inferior vena cava and the gallbladder fossa. The middle hepatic vein runs within this fissure. The right segmental fissure divides the front and back parts of the right lobe of the liver. The front and back segments of the right portal vein run to the middle of each of these parts. The right hepatic vein also runs within this fissure.

The left segmental fissure divides the middle and sides of the left lobe of the liver. The left intersegmental fissure delineates the top, middle, and bottom divisions of the left lobe of the liver.

Copyright © Mometrix Media. You have been licensed one copy of this document for personal use only. Any other reproduction or redistribution is strictly prohibited. All rights reserved.
This content is provided for test preparation purposes only and does not imply an endorsement by Mometrix of any particular political, scientific, or religious point of view.

The ligamentum teres runs along the outer edge of the falciform ligament. The middle-third-of-left-intersegmental fissure runs along the front side of the caudate lobe.

Congenital Abnormalities of the Liver

Congenital abnormalities of the liver are very rare and account for less than five percent of structural abnormalities.

The possibility of a congenital abnormality should be kept in mind when an unexplained mass is encountered.

One of the most well known (of these types of abnormalities) is called Riedel's lobe. This is a triangular-shaped projection (with the base of the triangle attached to the right lobe of the liver). It is usually located towards the front of the right lobe of the liver and is more common in women than men.

Other types of congenital abnormalities of the liver include:

- Absence of one or more of its lobes.
- Deformed lobes
- Decreased size of the lobes (In a normal liver, the right lobe is much larger than the left)
- Transposition of the gallbladder

Four Fossae of the Liver

The left sagittal fossa is a deep groove that extends from the notch on the front of the liver to the upper border of the back. It forms a separation between the right and left lobes.

The fossa for the umbilical vein provides space for the umbilical vein in the fetus. In the adult, it takes the form of the ligamentum teres (or round ligament) and is positioned between the quadrate lobe and the left lobe of the liver.

The fossa for the gallbladder is a shallow "deflated balloon" shaped groove that provides space under right lobe of the liver for the gallbladder and the cystic duct.

The fossa for the inferior vena cava is a short, deep cylindrical-shaped cut out that provides space for the vena cava. It extends upward and is located between the caudate lobe and the bare area of the liver.

Functions of the Liver

The liver is responsible for performing many vital functions in the body including:

- Production of bile
- Production of certain blood plasma proteins
- Production of cholesterol (and certain proteins needed to carry fats)
- Storage of excess glucose in the form of glycogen (that can be converted back to glucose when needed)
- Regulation of amino acids.
- Processing of hemoglobin (to store iron)
- Conversion of ammonia (that is poisonous to the body) to urea (a waste product excreted in urine)
- Purification of the blood (clears out drugs and other toxins)

Copyright © Mometrix Media. You have been licensed one copy of this document for personal use only. Any other reproduction or redistribution is strictly prohibited. All rights reserved.
This content is provided for test preparation purposes only and does not imply an endorsement by Mometrix of any particular political, scientific, or religious point of view.

- Regulation of blood clotting
- Controlling infections by boosting immune factors and removing bacteria.

The liver processes all of the blood that passes through the digestive system. The nutrients (and drugs) that pass through the liver are converted into forms that are appropriate for the body to use.

Transplanted Organs

Liver Transplants

Postoperative Complications

When evaluating a patient that is status post liver transplant, there are several complications that the vascular technologist should evaluate for. It is especially concerning when liver function tests are abnormal postoperatively, and the vascular technologist will be evaluating the liver vasculature for signs of thrombosis, stenosis, or the development of pseudoaneurysms. This evaluation is completed with gray-scale, color, and pulsed-wave Doppler evaluation of the major vessels of the liver and those that supply and drain the digestive system. It is also necessary to evaluate the IVC. If the patient is having pain, nausea, vomiting, or has a fever, it is important to check for perihepatic fluid collections, which may indicate seromas or hematomas, abscesses, or narrowing and/or dilation of the bile ducts.

Evaluating Patients

A follow-up ultrasound will typically be ordered within the first 24 hours after a patient has undergone surgery for a liver transplant because early awareness of complications may decrease the likelihood of transplant failure. The basic protocol is to evaluate the entire abdomen to check for any fluid collections and any signs of pancreatitis. The liver is evaluated with gray-scale, color, and spectral Doppler. Gray-scale imaging is important for determining the size, echogenicity, and texture of the liver. Gray-scale imaging can also be used to initially check the vessels of the liver as well and measure the diameter of the portal vein and to check for any dilation of the bile ducts. Color and spectral Doppler provide important information regarding patency and the direction of blood flow and to evaluate for any turbulence within the main portal vein and its intrahepatic branches, the hepatic veins, and the main hepatic artery as well as its intrahepatic arterial branches and the IVC. It is important to evaluate the anastomoses as well. The PSV, resistive index (RI), and acceleration time measurements should be calculated during spectral Doppler interrogation with special attention given to angle correction.

Kidney Transplants

Scanning the Transplanted Kidney

Select a transducer with the highest frequency for depth penetration, usually a 5-MHz one is adequate. A curved transducer gives a large field allowing for accurate length measurements of the entire kidney. Using the postoperative scar helps to locate the transplanted kidney. Long axis views of the kidney will appear along the axis of the scar and the transverse view of the kidney will be at a right angle to the scar. The urinary bladder will be scanned. If the bladder is full of urine, voiding may make what appears as hydronephrosis disappear when scanned again. Color Doppler may be helpful to image flow of blood to and from the transplanted kidney.

Copyright © Mometrix Media. You have been licensed one copy of this document for personal use only. Any other reproduction or redistribution is strictly prohibited. All rights reserved.
This content is provided for test preparation purposes only and does not imply an endorsement by Mometrix of any particular political, scientific, or religious point of view.

Functions of the Kidneys and Urinary Tract

Following are the major functions of the kidneys and urinary tract:

- **Toxin Removal**: The human body is constantly accumulating toxins either from food digestion or waste products produced by cells. These toxins need to be removed quickly or they will build up to dangerous levels in the blood. The kidneys filter the toxins out of the blood and safely eliminate them for the body in the form of urine.
- **Drug Removal**: Many drugs are eliminated in the urine after being metabolized.
- **Maintaining a proper fluid balance**: The body is constantly gaining fluid (from the diet) and losing it (evaporation, urine, stool). The kidneys regulate the body's fluid balance to keep it from swelling up or becoming dehydrated.
- **Electrolyte Balance**: In order for cells to function properly, the concentrations of electrolytes in the blood need to be tightly controlled. The kidneys regulate this process. Here are the most important electrolytes and the organs that are sensitive to their changes:
    - Sodium – Brain and nerves
    - Potassium, Magnesium – Heart, muscle, and nerves
    - Calcium – Heart, muscle, nerves, and bone
    - Phosphorus – Muscle and bone
- **Acid-Base Balance**: The body's processing of proteins is sensitive to changes in acid concentration of blood. The kidneys remove excess acid to maintain the proper pH balance.
- **Blood Pressure Control**: The kidneys play a role in regulating blood pressure by balancing fluid and salt levels in the blood.
- **Hormone Production**: The kidneys produce erythropoietin (affects the bone marrow to make more red blood cells) and calcitriol (active form of vitamin D for bone health)

Kidney Stones

Kidney stones (renal calculi) are solid crystals made up of dissolved minerals that occur in urine. They are typically found inside the kidneys or ureters. The size of the stone can be as large as a golf ball. Tiny kidney stones usually leave the body in the urine stream unnoticed. The larger stones can cause an obstruction of a ureter. This in turn causes the ureter to swell with urine and causes moderate to severe pain. The pain is most commonly felt in the back (flank), lower abdomen, and groin. The most common composition of kidney stones is calcium oxalate.

Clinical symptoms of kidney stones include intermittent back (flank) pain, vomiting, red blood cells in the urine (hematuria), infection, and an elevated white blood cell (leukocyte) count.

Ultrasound Both Right and Left Kidneys

The right kidney is best seen if the sonographer has the patient lie supine and the transducer is angled obliquely. The liver acts as the window for the sound beam. A coronal and a lateral approach are also possible. It is often helpful to have the patient roll to a right-side-up position and the transducer used at a lateral approach. To scan the left kidney, have the patient left-side up. The patient raises the arm above his head and the technician uses the coronal approach to scan through the spleen. Using the transducer at a decubitus and oblique position look for the clearest image of the left kidney with the highest frequency available. Use pillows under the patient to eliminate the cavity between the ribs and the hip bone.

Solitary Kidney

A solitary kidney is a rare condition. It occurs when only one kidney is formed (instead of two) during embryonic development due to agenesis (the absence or failed development of a body part).

Copyright © Mometrix Media. You have been licensed one copy of this document for personal use only. Any other reproduction or redistribution is strictly prohibited. All rights reserved.
This content is provided for test preparation purposes only and does not imply an endorsement by Mometrix of any particular political, scientific, or religious point of view.

The solitary functioning kidney is typically enlarged, and the remaining "empty" kidney location should be examined for the presence of a small, non-functional kidney.

Pelvic Kidney

If a kidney is not observed in its normal location, the patient's retroperitoneum and pelvis should be scanned. In most cases the "lost" kidney will be found in the patient's bony pelvis region. Pelvic kidney is a developmental abnormality in which the kidney (or kidneys) is located in pelvis instead of normal abdominal lumbar position in the renal fossa.

Anatomy of the Kidneys

- Blood is supplied to the kidneys by the renal artery. The renal artery originates from the aorta.
- The renal artery splits into three branches as it enters the kidney through the hilus. Two of these branches are located in front of the ureter and one is located behind the pelvis of the ureter.
- A total of five to six veins join together to form the renal vein. The renal vein exits the hilus directly in front of the renal artery and drains into the inferior vena cava (IVC).
- The lymph vessels run along the renal artery and join the lateral aortic lymph nodes (near the origin of the renal artery).
- Nerves line the branches of the renal vessels and begin in the renal sympathetic plexus.

Anatomy of the Kidneys and Urinary Tract

The kidneys are two dark-red bean-shaped organs located at the back of the abdominal cavity just below the ribs (one on each side of the spine). Each kidney is about four inches long and two inches thick. There is an adrenal gland located above each kidney. The kidneys lie under the peritoneum in a cushion of two types of fat (perirenal and pararenal). The right kidney typically lies lower than the left due to the presence of the liver.

Blood is supplied to the kidneys via two renal arteries (that branch off of the abdominal aorta). Blood leaves the kidneys through the renal veins.

The urinary tract is made up of a series of organs that produce, store, and eliminate urine. It is composed of two kidneys, two ureters, the urinary bladder, two sphincter muscles and the urethra.

Horseshoe Kidneys

Horseshoe kidneys are the most common congenital fusion abnormality and are often an incidental diagnosis. People with horseshoe kidneys can lead a normal life, but it is important to diagnose horseshoe kidneys prior to any abdominal surgery because the anatomy can vary so it is important for the surgical team to be aware of this condition. Also, for anybody that needs renal imaging or procedures to be performed, it is imperative to be aware of this anomaly beforehand because it is not uncommon to have multiple renal arteries with horseshoe kidneys. A patient with horseshoe kidneys demonstrates a lower lying position of the kidneys that are positioned near the middle of the body. Horseshoe kidneys are typically fused at the lower poles, which tend to be directed in a more medial position. Although some individuals don't have any issues at all, others will be prone

Copyright © Mometrix Media. You have been licensed one copy of this document for personal use only. Any other reproduction or redistribution is strictly prohibited. All rights reserved.
This content is provided for test preparation purposes only and does not imply an endorsement by Mometrix of any particular political, scientific, or religious point of view.

to kidney stones, hydronephrosis, or urinary tract infections. The diagram demonstrates horseshoe kidneys that are fused at the lower poles.

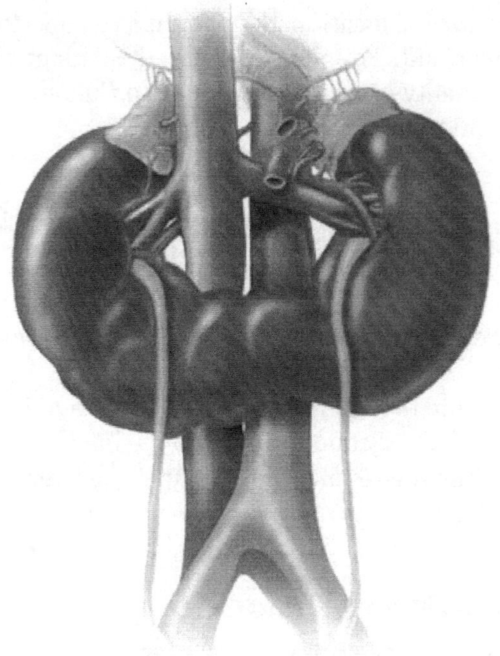

Renal Transplants

Preferred Location

Most renal transplants are implanted in the iliac fossa of the recipient, with the right iliac fossa being the preferred location. Typically, the left kidney of the donor is removed because the length of the left renal vein is longer than the right. The left kidney is then rotated and implanted into the right iliac fossa. This region is used because it does not interfere with any of the abdominal or pelvic organs, and it is in close proximity to the urinary bladder, which will allow a shorter segment of the ureter to be used and still be inserted above the point at which the native ureter enters the urinary bladder. The iliac fossa is also close to the blood vessels of the iliac region such as the external iliac vein and the internal iliac artery as the transplanted artery needs. Also, this location does not require the removal of the native kidney, which means less risk of infection.

Postoperative Evaluation

It is important for the vascular technologist to look at the patient's medical records in order to determine the approach that should be used for the anastomosis used during his or her renal transplant, and, when available, comparisons should always be made to any prior exams. If the surgery is performed as a live-donor renal transplant, typically the graft of the renal artery will be connected end to end with the internal iliac artery or an end-to-side anastomosis will be formed with the external iliac artery. When the kidney is harvested from a cadaver, the main renal artery is removed with part of the aorta to create an end-to-side connection to the external iliac artery of the recipient. An end-to-side anastomosis approach is the most frequently used connection of the renal vein to the external iliac vein. The ureter of the donor usually enters the dome of the urinary bladder, although sometimes it may be necessary to use the ureter of the recipient. Notably, if the

Copyright © Mometrix Media. You have been licensed one copy of this document for personal use only. Any other reproduction or redistribution is strictly prohibited. All rights reserved.
This content is provided for test preparation purposes only and does not imply an endorsement by Mometrix of any particular political, scientific, or religious point of view.

cadaver donor is younger than five years old, both of the kidneys may be implanted into the same recipient.

Diagnosing Rejection

Many physicians rely on a renal biopsy to diagnose rejection of the transplanted kidney. However, when a sonogram is ordered to evaluate for rejection of the transplant, the vascular technologist should use gray-scale ultrasound to measure the maximum size of the kidney in the longitudinal and transverse planes. Any fluid collections should also be documented if present. It is important to compare the results of this study with any previous ultrasounds that have been performed to determine if there is an increase in size. The echogenicity of the cortex of the transplanted kidney should also be evaluated to determine if it is more echogenic, which is also an indication of rejection. The transplanted kidney should also be evaluated for signs of hydronephrosis, and documentation of the level of obstruction should be determined, if possible. Duplex scanning can be used to provide information about complications such as thrombosis of the renal vein, stenosis of the renal artery, and if an AVF has occurred. Some labs will measure the resistivity index to determine an acute rejection, but this is not widely accepted.

Non-Removal of Kidneys

Kidney transplants do not typically require the removal of the patient's native kidneys. If the kidneys do not need to be removed, this may mean an easier recovery for the patient. It can take up to eight weeks for a patient to recover when the native kidneys must be taken out, and more incisions increase the risk of infection. Another concern of removing the native kidneys is the necessity of a blood transfusion because this may prompt antibodies to form, which could be a detriment to the transplanted kidney, but these concerns are decreased if the native kidneys need to be removed after the transplant. The native kidneys are not usually removed unless the patient has cancer or polycystic kidneys, which creates an enlargement of the kidneys due to the multiple cysts.

Effect of Portal Hypertension on the Spleen

Portal hypertension is the buildup of pressure in the portal vein (the vein connecting the intestines and the liver). Normally, the pressure is low compared with the arterial pressure, but slightly above the pressure in the other veins of the body. The most common cause of portal hypertension is liver disease (such as cirrhosis). Portal hypertension usually causes moderate splenomegality and dilated, tortuous blood vessels at the splenic hilum. It also causes dilation of the portal vein itself. If portal hypertension is suspected, the liver and portal vein should be examined along with the spleen.

Spleen

The spleen is in the upper left of the abdomen. It is located behind the stomach and immediately below the diaphragm. It is about the size of a thick paperback book and weighs just over half a pound. It is made up of lymphoid tissue. The blood vessels are connected to the spleen by splenic sinuses (modified capillaries). The following peritoneal ligaments support the spleen:

- The gastrolienal ligament that connects the stomach to the spleen.
- The lienorenal ligament that connects the kidney to the spleen.
- The middle section of the phrenicocolic ligament (connects the left colic flexure to the thoracic diaphragm).

The main functions of the spleen are to filter unwanted materials from the blood (including old red blood cells) and to help fight infections.

Copyright © Mometrix Media. You have been licensed one copy of this document for personal use only. Any other reproduction or redistribution is strictly prohibited. All rights reserved.
This content is provided for test preparation purposes only and does not imply an endorsement by Mometrix of any particular political, scientific, or religious point of view.

Up to ten percent of the population has one or more accessory spleens that tend to form at the hilum of the original spleen.

Calculating the Volume of a Patient's Spleen

One of the advantages of sonography is quickly being able to measure organs or other anatomical structures within the body. These measurements are useful in the follow-up treatment of many diseases. These measurements can be added to and displayed on a calculations worksheet for the physician that will be interpreting the results. When it is necessary to calculate the volume of an organ, the user will measure the spleen (in this example) in three planes using 2D ultrasound. Volume is displayed in any units of length cubed and is calculated by multiplying the length times the width times the height. Organs are typically measured in centimeters; therefore, the volume is in centimeters cubed (cm^3). Three-dimensional ultrasound is also used to calculate the volume of an organ. This method is actually considered to be superior to measurements obtained on 2D images, but it requires more time to perform.

Trauma to the Spleen

Blunt abdominal trauma is the most common reason for injury to the spleen. Motor vehicle accidents are the primary cause (accounting for up to thirty percent of cases). Additionally, any of the diseases (such as portal hypertension) that cause splenic enlargement may cause the spleen to rupture. The affected patient usually presents with upper left quadrant pain. Hypotension and a decreased hemoglobin level may indicate internal bleeding.

The following ultrasound features are present:

- Splenomegaly with progressive enlargement and an irregular splenic border.
- Focal hematomas are represented by intrasplenic fluid collections.
- Sub-capsular hematomas show perispleic fluid collections.
- Blood exhibits various echo patterns (depending on the age of the injury).
- Focal areas show tiny lacerations that give rise to small collections of blood interspersed with disrupted pulp (contusion).
- When the spleen heals (and returns to normal) small, irregular foci may remain.

Infarction of the Spleen

Infarction of the spleen is usually caused by infection or a blood clot. Several conditions that may cause infarction of the spleen include pancreatitis, endocarditis, leukemia/lymphoma, and sickle cell anemia. Its ultrasound appearance is dependent on when the infarct occurs. A fresh infarct (hemorrhagic) appears hypoechoic. A healed infarct (with scarring) appears as an echogenic, wedge-shaped lesion. The affected patient will usually present with pain in the upper left quadrant of the abdomen. Additional symptoms may include fever, chills, nausea, vomiting, chest pain (upon breathing), and left shoulder pain. Splenic abscess may result, especially if the infarct was caused by an infection.

Effect of Histoplasmosis on the Spleen

Histoplasmosis is a disease caused by the fungus histoplasma capsulatum (a common soil-based fungus found in the central and eastern U.S.). The disease primarily affects the lungs (since the dry fungal spores are usually inhaled). The symptoms are similar to tuberculosis. It can, however affect other organs in the body. This form of the disease is called disseminated histoplasmosis, and it can be fatal (especially if left untreated). Disseminated histoplasmosis is more frequently seen in patients with cancer or AIDS. Using ultrasound, the affected spleen appears with multiple focal, bright, echogenic, granulomatous lesions throughout.

Copyright © Mometrix Media. You have been licensed one copy of this document for personal use only. Any other reproduction or redistribution is strictly prohibited. All rights reserved.
This content is provided for test preparation purposes only and does not imply an endorsement by Mometrix of any particular political, scientific, or religious point of view.

Cysts of the Spleen

Eighty percent of all splenic cysts are pseudocysts (an abnormal structure that resembles a cyst but has no membranous lining). They are usually the result of prior trauma to the spleen. More rarely, they can also be caused by congenital conditions (epidermoid cysts) and parasites (echinococcal). Affected patients typically present with a symptom-free lower upper quadrant mass.

The following ultrasound features are present:

- Parasitic cysts appear as anechoic lesions (with possible calcification) or as solid masses (with fine internal echoes and poor distal enhancement).
- True (or primary cysts) are typically solitary and rarely calcified.
- Both types of cysts have well defined walls.

Benign Tumors of the Spleen

There are three main types of benign tumors that affect the spleen. They are:

- Hamartomas: A common benign tumor of the spleen composed of splenic tissue that grows in a disorganized mass. They are usually asymptomatic. On ultrasound, they appear as well-defined hyperechoic solid masses.
- Cavernous hemangiomas: These tumors are made up jumbled growths of blood vessels fed by numerous tributary arteries. They typically go through a growth phase followed by a rest phase (during which they virtually disappear). They only cause symptoms if they bleed or increase the size of the spleen enough to affect other organs. On ultrasound, they usually appear as a large echogenic mass with small hypoechoic areas.
- Cystic lymphangiomas: A rare benign congenital tumor. It appears as a mass with extensive cystic replacement of the normal splenic tissue.

Malignant Tumors of the Spleen

There are three main types of cancerous tumors that affect the spleen. They are:

- Hemangiosarcoma: This is an aggressive form of cancer. It is a blood-fed sarcoma (the blood vessels grow directly into the tumor and it is typically filled with blood). A frequent cause of death is the rupture of the tumor (which causes severe bleeding). On ultrasound, the tumor has a mixed cystic pattern.
- Lymphoma: Any of the various malignant tumors (of lymphatic and reticuloendothelial tissues) that occur as circumscribed solid tumors. They are composed of cells that resemble lymphocytes, plasma cells, or histiocytes.
- Metastases: Cancer that has spread from other organs of the body. The spleen is the tenth most common site for this type of cancer. It appears (on ultrasound) as multiple, hyperechoic lesions.

Anatomic Variants Visualized When Scanning the Spleen

If the sonographer visualizes a mass located in the splenic hilum, an accessory spleen must be considered. It is a common variant that is a congenital anomaly, and it can be identified as an oval or spherical "mass" that has the same appearance as the tissue found in the spleen. Although the typical location is within the splenic hilum, it may actually be visualized anywhere in the abdominal or pelvic cavity. A wandering spleen occurs when this organ is not in the usual left upper quadrant (LUQ) location. The ligaments that typically hold the spleen in place were not present at birth, which may allow the spleen to migrate from the LUQ. If this occurs, the vessels of the spleen may become twisted and cut off blood supply to it. Another variant includes the shape of the spleen,

Copyright © Mometrix Media. You have been licensed one copy of this document for personal use only. Any other reproduction or redistribution is strictly prohibited. All rights reserved.
This content is provided for test preparation purposes only and does not imply an endorsement by Mometrix of any particular political, scientific, or religious point of view.

which can look different from patient to patient and not take on the typical elliptical shape with a concave border inferiorly.

Appearance of an Enlarged Lymph Node

During various ultrasound exams, a vascular technologist may discover enlarged lymph nodes throughout the body. These lymph nodes are often visualized in the neck, axilla, and groin and may be an incidental finding. Enlarged lymph nodes may be related to cancers such as lymphoma or to inflammation within the body. A normal lymph node takes on an oval or elliptical shape with a central hilum that is hyperechoic. A hypoechoic area will surround the hilum. When using color Doppler, the hilum will demonstrate some blood flow, but in a lymph node that is enlarged there is a lot of blood flow and the node itself tends to take on a more circular shape.

Implanted Ventricular Assist Device

If an individual has been diagnosed with heart failure, he or she may be treated with a mechanism known as a ventricular assist device. If a patient has had a ventricular assist device implanted, the vascular technologist can expect to see flow patterns that are modified from what is typically seen. The flow patterns can differ based on which ventricular assist device is used. The most common apparatus used is the left ventricular assist device, which results in a nonpulsatile spectral waveform because continuous flow pumps are used. The PSV and EDV will not be measured due to the nonpulsatility. One end of the device is affixed to the left ventricle with the other end attached to the aorta. If the patient has a biventricular assist device, the spectral analysis will depend on if the flow pump is continuous or pulsatile, which can severely underestimate PSVs.

Copyright © Mometrix Media. You have been licensed one copy of this document for personal use only. Any other reproduction or redistribution is strictly prohibited. All rights reserved.
This content is provided for test preparation purposes only and does not imply an endorsement by Mometrix of any particular political, scientific, or religious point of view.

Arterial Peripheral Vasculature

Effect of Making a Fist on the Waveform of the Brachial Artery

If a patient is asked to make a fist during an upper extremity Doppler exam, the waveform of the brachial artery will likely appear more pulsatile, which, in turn, results in a higher pulsatility index. Recall that the pulsatility index offers quantitative information and can be calculated by the following formula: $\frac{\text{PS}-\text{ED}}{\text{mean}}$, where PS is the peak-systolic velocity, ED is the end-diastolic velocity, and mean represents the mean velocity. Typically, less distal resistance will demonstrate a waveform with low pulsatility, and high resistance will demonstrate a waveform that has increased pulsatility. Having the patient make a fist will create more resistance in the arteries that are found in a more distal location of the upper extremity, and the vascular technologist will also notice that the amount of diastolic blood flow has likely been reduced.

Blood Flow After It Reaches the Brachial Artery

The brachial artery is found in the upper arm and is used to determine an individual's blood pressure. The brachial artery receives blood flow from the axillary artery and carries it to the antecubital fossa, which is located in the anterior region of the arm where the elbow bends. It is in this region that the brachial artery branches into the radial and ulnar arteries. The radial artery is found on the same side as one of the bones of the forearm known as the radius (located on the lateral or thumb side). The ulnar artery is the other branch that stems from the brachial artery and is found on the medial (pinkie) side of the forearm. The radial and ulnar arteries supply the hand with the necessary blood flow.

Spectral Waveform Seen in a Normal Brachial Artery

When a vascular technologist is interrogating the arteries of the upper extremities with spectral Doppler, it is important to note that the waveform of the brachial artery should display high resistance. This is because it is a peripheral artery with smaller distal arterioles that impedes the blood flow from arteries to the more distal arterioles. Depending on the age of the patient, normal waveforms of the brachial artery will demonstrate a triphasic or biphasic waveform. As people age, elasticity is lost in the blood vessels, which can result in a more biphasic flow. In younger individuals, a short reversal of flow will be demonstrated at the end of systole and then the blood flows forward once again. This triphasic waveform also demonstrates a brisk upstroke and downstroke during systole.

Participate in Manual Compression of Pseudoaneurysms

More radiographic procedures are being performed, which translates to more pseudoaneurysm formation, especially of the CFA. Ultrasound can be used to diagnose this condition, but it can also be used as a guide during compression. The size of the aneurysm should be documented along with the diameter of the neck. Gray-scale and color Doppler should be used to make sure that the transducer is compressing the neck so blood cannot move into the sac while still enabling the blood to flow into the femoral artery. This compression should take roughly 10 to 20 minutes, and it can be applied with the ultrasound transducer. After this time frame, the pressure can be released to see if there has been clotting of the pseudoaneurysm.

Blood Flow from the Popliteal Artery

The femoral artery of the thigh extends through an area known as the adductor (Hunter's) canal and becomes the popliteal artery in the region of the posterior knee. The popliteal artery is a relatively short blood vessel that supplies oxygenated blood to the knee and surrounding tissues. Although this blood vessel tends to be very short, it does have branches to supply the skin and

Copyright © Mometrix Media. You have been licensed one copy of this document for personal use only. Any other reproduction or redistribution is strictly prohibited. All rights reserved.
This content is provided for test preparation purposes only and does not imply an endorsement by Mometrix of any particular political, scientific, or religious point of view.

muscles, which can serve as collateral vessels in cases of obstruction. The first vessel to stem from the popliteal artery is the anterior tibial artery, which supplies oxygenated blood to the lower leg and foot. The popliteal artery also branches into the tibioperoneal trunk, which gives off several branches to also supply blood to the lower leg and foot.

Claudication

Claudication is pain in the extremities due to narrowing of the aorta or peripheral arteries, which is called peripheral arterial disease (PAD). Atherosclerosis is often the cause of claudication, which results in decreased blood flow to the extremities, especially during exercise. In the early stages, patients may describe their symptoms as pain or aching that often disappears during rest. As the narrowing of the vessels increases, patients may complain of pain even when resting. Other symptoms may include weakness of the limbs, skin discoloration and/or ulcers, or cold feet. The lower extremities are affected more often than the arms. The vessels that exhibit atherosclerosis or arteriosclerosis are the femoral and popliteal arteries. Blockages can develop in the aorta and iliac vessels as well.

Claudication Location Symptoms

When patients experience claudication, the location of symptoms can often determine at which level the diseased arteries are located. For example, if the patient has pain on both sides of the buttocks, then it is assumed that there is significant disease of the distal aorta and or iliac arteries. If only one side is symptomatic, then unilateral iliofemoral disease is suspected of the ipsilateral (same) side.

Location of claudication symptoms	Type of disease present	Unilateral symptoms
Buttocks	Aortoiliac disease when pain is bilateral	The iliofemoral region is suspected when pain is unilateral.
Thigh	Distal external iliac/common femoral	This could be a unilateral finding.
Calf	Femoral/popliteal	This could be a unilateral finding.

Segmental Doppler Pressure

Physicians will order a segmental Doppler pressure as a screening exam to evaluate issues that the patient has with circulation. Segmental pressures are commonly ordered because they are a noninvasive exam to assess the blood flow within the arteries of the extremities. This test can help determine if PAD is present, and in patients that have known PAD, the advancement of the disease can be tracked and compared with prior studies. Segmental Doppler pressures can also help determine if an artery is diseased (and can provide clues to the approximate location), and they can also be used to determine any surgical treatments that may be necessary such as bypass grafting. As a screening exam, segmental pressures will provide clues as to whether an artery is stenosed or occluded (although it cannot discern between the two).

Inflating the Blood Pressure Cuff

During Doppler pressure exams, the vascular technologist should start by taking bilateral brachial arterial pressures and documenting both readings. The vascular technologist must remember the highest brachial pressure reading because this value will be used not only to calculate the ABIs, but also when taking other pressure measurements. For example, the cuff should be inflated 20–30 mmHg more than the highest brachial arterial systolic pressure. Once the arterial Doppler sound is no longer heard, the vascular technologist should continue to increase the blood pressure cuff

Copyright © Mometrix Media. You have been licensed one copy of this document for personal use only. Any other reproduction or redistribution is strictly prohibited. All rights reserved.
This content is provided for test preparation purposes only and does not imply an endorsement by Mometrix of any particular political, scientific, or religious point of view.

pressure 20–30 mmHg higher than this point. If it is determined that the pressures must be repeated, the sonographer should wait for roughly a minute after deflation of the cuff to allow the blood flow to return to the artery because if the next pressure reading is taken too soon, it could be miscalculated at a value lower than the actual reading.

Vascular technologists must consider the size of blood pressure cuffs that are chosen for each patient and the area of the extremities used for pressure readings. Vascular labs will typically have their chosen protocols regarding the number of cuffs that are used (either the three- or four-cuff methods). When performing pressure measurements of the upper extremities, there will typically be three cuffs that are applied to the wrist, forearm, and upper arm. The wrist cuff used is usually 5–10 cm, the forearm cuff chosen will usually be a 10 cm cuff, with a 12 cm cuff being selected for the upper arm. Exams of the lower extremities may either be three- or four-cuff techniques with the ankle and calf level using a 10 cm cuff, if a three-cuff method is used, a 17–19 cm cuff is applied to the thigh, and if a four-cuff method is chosen, then the sonographer should select a 12 cm for the upper and lower region of the thigh.

Obtaining Segmental Pressures

When a patient is having a segmental pressure exam, it is important to have the patient lie on the ultrasound table in a supine position. A pillow should be offered to the patient (and the head of the bed can be raised just slightly if the patient is uncomfortable with just a pillow), but the goal is to have the heart and extremities in the same plane. The patient should be instructed to relax the legs so they are straight, and the arms should be down by the sides. The reason that the heart and extremities should be in roughly the same plane with the patient supine is to overcome the response to hydrostatic pressure because the pressure of the ankle increases when the patient stands because it depends on the distance of the artery from the heart as well as the force of gravity. As long as the patient is supine, there is only a slight effect of hydrostatic pressure witnessed within the arteries and veins.

Cuff Artifacts

While performing segmental pressures, sonographers must take extra care in choosing the size of the cuff for each patient and the size of their extremities in order to avoid cuff artifact. A cuff artifact can lead to a misdiagnosis of the patient because it can mistakenly create pressures that are either too high or too low. The width of the cuff should be at least 20% greater than the patient's extremity. If the cuff is not wide enough, for example, during a lower extremity exam, it could result in a pressure reading that is higher than it should be. If the cuff is too large, then a low-pressure reading will likely occur. If a four-cuff method is used, it is important to note that if a cuff artifact is present it is usually found in the high thigh with the pressure being 30 mmHg greater than the brachial arterial pressure that was found to be a higher value.

Normal Peripheral Venous vs. Arterial Waveforms

The venous system returns oxygen back to the right atrium of the heart. The blood from the lower extremities returns to the heart via the IVC. The pressure within the venous system is much lower than the pressure found in the arterial system, and when interrogating peripheral veins above the knee with spectral Doppler, it should demonstrate spontaneous flow. Spontaneous blood flow confirms that the vessel is not obstructed. The venous waveform should be phasic when the patient inhales and exhales. The blood in the arterial system is transferred out of the heart and delivered to all of the body's cells. The spectral waveform of the peripheral arteries will typically exhibit blood flow that has high resistance and is either biphasic or triphasic with bidirectional flow. If a patient presents with narrowing of the arteries, the waveform tends to demonstrate continuous flow in only one direction with decreased resistance.

Copyright © Mometrix Media. You have been licensed one copy of this document for personal use only. Any other reproduction or redistribution is strictly prohibited. All rights reserved.
This content is provided for test preparation purposes only and does not imply an endorsement by Mometrix of any particular political, scientific, or religious point of view.

Ankle-Brachial Index

An ankle-brachial index (ABI) is often one of the first tests performed to help screen for PAD when clinically indicated and the findings can help physicians determine if it is mild or severe. These indices are calculated to determine if there is a drop of pressure distal to an artery that is significantly stenosed and is a ratio that compares the blood pressure findings of the lower extremities to the body's overall blood pressure (also referred to as the systemic blood pressure). For ABI calculations, various systolic pressures are recorded in multiple arteries of the lower extremities and the highest arterial pressure on one side of the ankle will be divided by the highest arterial pressure from the highest measurement of the brachial artery. Although it doesn't tell clinicians exactly where the stenosis or occlusion is, it can help narrow down the location.

In order to calculate the ABI, the vascular technologist will first obtain bilateral brachial pressures of the arms. The pressure reading that is the highest will be used later to calculate the ABI value. Two pressures within the ankle are also taken, and the highest reading will be used to calculate the ABI. The two arteries that are used in the ankle region are the DPA and the PTA. Once the pressures are obtained on each side, the vascular technologist may calculate the ABI by taking the highest pressure reading of either the DPA or PTA and dividing it by the highest brachial pressure of either the right or left arm.

Calculating the ABI in the Calf

To determine the ABI, the vascular technologist will record the pressures at the ankle level of the PTA as well as the DPA. An ABI is calculated separately for the PTA and DPA by dividing these pressures by the highest brachial arterial pressure that was recorded from both arms. However, the highest calculated ABI will be calculated and used for each side. An ABI will be calculated bilaterally for comparison. Notably, ankle pressures are typically equal to or greater than the blood pressure reading of the brachial artery that is the highest. When performing lower extremity exams, the pressure measurements should be performed in the distal leg first and then moved proximally.

Obtaining Segmental Pressures

When a patient describes symptoms of claudication, but the segmental pressure exam is within normal limits (or when the results are borderline normal), then protocols typically involve having the patient exercise whenever possible. Another reason that patients are required to exercise is if they have already been diagnosed with arterial disease but the extent of the disease during exercise has not yet been determined. The vascular technologist will typically calculate ABIs first without exercise. Immediately after the patient stops exercising, ABIs are calculated every two minutes until the results are restored to the numbers calculated before the patient walked on the treadmill. If the patient is unable to walk on the treadmill, it is possible to have them perform toe raises during the exercise phase.

Claudication and Cardiac Treadmill Exercise Exams

Regardless of the type of exercise exams performed, it is important for the sonographer to closely monitor the patient and his or her blood pressure. When the patient is required to exercise for symptoms of claudication, he or she will be asked to walk on a treadmill until the pain becomes unbearable or for no more than five minutes. The treadmill is usually set with an incline of 12%, and the speed will be between 1.5 and 2 mph (2 mph is preferred), but once the speed is set it does not typically change. The goal of cardiac treadmill exercise testing is to achieve a target heart rate that is determined for this patient, which can be achieved by increasing the incline and speed of the treadmill during various times throughout the study.

Copyright © Mometrix Media. You have been licensed one copy of this document for personal use only. Any other reproduction or redistribution is strictly prohibited. All rights reserved.
This content is provided for test preparation purposes only and does not imply an endorsement by Mometrix of any particular political, scientific, or religious point of view.

Time of Recovery and Diagnosis

If the patient is asked to exercise, the vascular technologist has already performed pre-exercise testing ABIs and pressure readings. Post-exercise testing ABIs and pressures are attained right after the patient is done exercising and then at two-minute intervals until the pre-exercise values are reached. Determination of a single level or more than one level can be discerned by comparing the pre- and postexercise values. If the patient's pressures reach the pre-exercise numbers in less than 5 minutes, this suggests that the patient only has disease in one level. Disease in more than one level is suggested when it takes more than 12 minutes for the pre-exercise levels to be reached. Normal post-exercise findings include an increase of the ABIs and the pressure values. If the pressure readings fall below those that were obtained while the patient was at rest, it suggests that disease is present, with more significant disease equating to a greater decline in pressure readings.

Effect of Exercise on Peripheral Arteries

Peripheral resistance is a common term that is discussed in vascular ultrasound. As arteries extend in a more distal location, they typically become smaller in diameter as they approach the terminal arterioles. This decrease in the diameter of the blood vessels increases the resistance of blood that is moving within the peripheral arteries. Exercise will enable vasodilation within the smaller vessels, which will decrease the amount of peripheral resistance so that more blood can reach the skeletal muscles, which is a requirement during exercise. Flow reversal in a spectral Doppler waveform will be decreased, and the signal becomes one that demonstrates low resistance during exercise.

Peripheral Resistance and the Pulse Amplitude

An arterial pressure wave is the typical type of energy that is created when blood is flowing in the human body. As blood is pumped out of the heart, the arteries become distended, but the arterioles do not respond with the same amount of distension. Because of the lack of elastin in the arterioles, in diastole the pressure energy is converted to kinetic energy. When vasoconstriction takes place, the peripheral resistance increases distally and a greater amount of the pressure energy in the proximal portion of the arterial vessels will be reflected. This equates to an increase of the pulse amplitude of the arterial wave when it is added to the energy that is already present in the arteries that are in a more proximal location.

Hyperemia with and Without Arterial Obstruction

Hyperemia refers to an increased amount of blood flow to a limb (or any part of the body). If a patient experiences hyperemia in the presence of arterial obstruction, this condition tends to extend the amount of time that this occurs. In patients without a significant arterial obstruction, the hyperemia would take less time for the patient to recover after exercise. If the patient is unable to walk on the treadmill due to conditions such as breathing issues, heart problems, needs the assistance of a walker, or cannot walk for enough time to reproduce the symptoms that he or she has been having, then the reactive hyperemia technique may be used. This method should not be used, however, if the patient has a stent or a bypass graft because it requires the inflation of thigh cuffs to high levels creating too much pressure on the thigh.

Buerger's Disease

Buerger's disease, also referred to as thrombosis obliterans, is the most common type of arteritis. Arteritis occurs when the walls of the artery become inflamed, which can create a distal occlusion of the arteries within the fingers and toes due to a blood clot. Buerger's disease is almost always found in younger men between the ages of 20 and 40 that are heavy smokers or use chewing tobacco. It is assumed that the chemicals in cigarettes and chewing tobacco create swelling of the blood vessels.

Copyright © Mometrix Media. You have been licensed one copy of this document for personal use only. Any other reproduction or redistribution is strictly prohibited. All rights reserved.
This content is provided for test preparation purposes only and does not imply an endorsement by Mometrix of any particular political, scientific, or religious point of view.

Claudication is a common symptom that patients experience as well as numbness and/or tingling of the fingers or toes. The fingers or toes may have ulcers or gangrene, which can lead to their amputation.

Cause of Arterial Ulcers

When an individual experiences a decrease in perfusion to the lower extremities, there is an increased risk of development of an arterial ulcer. An ulcer occurs when there is a breakdown of skin and tissue in any area of the body. This opening can increase the risk of infection because bacteria can easily enter the wound. Arterial ulcers typically occur as a result of atherosclerosis, which hinders the blood supply to the limb, which exacerbates the amount of damage to the surrounding region. Arterial ulcerations, when compared to venous ulcers, tend to cause a great deal of pain. Antibiotics are often necessary, and prompt diagnosis and management are necessary to increase circulation to that area. The location of arterial ulcers often involves the lower extremity, especially the toes and sometimes near the tibia. Although these wounds don't bleed very often, they are frequently very deep, and the skin may have a shiny appearance.

Associated Embolus with a Peripheral Arterial Aneurysm

When a lower extremity develops a peripheral arterial aneurysm, there is often an associated thrombus within the lumen aneurysm. This thrombus forms because the blood inside the dilated vessel tends to take on a back-and-forth whirling configuration. When part of the clot breaks off, it often travels distally and lodges within a smaller digital artery. An embolus (emboli) can interrupt the transportation of blood distally to the individual's limb because it may become obstructed, creating what is known as blue toe syndrome. Although a rupture of an aneurysm of the abdominal aorta is the main concern, an embolism is the most common complication of a peripheral arterial aneurysm.

Emergency of Acute Occlusion

If an acute occlusion is suspected of the lower extremities, it is considered an emergency because oxygenated blood is not reaching the entire lower extremity, which may cause a loss of function of the extremities. For example, if the patient's mid femoral artery is occluded, everything distal to that blood vessel (the distal thigh, knee, lower leg, and foot) won't receive the blood that it should, which can cause ischemia or tissue death. This is a very serious condition that requires immediate treatment such as bypass, thrombolysis, or even embolectomy. Chronic arterial disease is not considered an emergency, on the other hand, because the longer an artery is stenosed, there has likely been ample time for collateral channels to form. Collateral pathways enable blood to be rerouted to bypass the area of the artery that is affected by the occlusion so the distal extremity can still be supplied with oxygenated blood.

Ischemic Rest Pain

Severe toe pain is an indication of ischemic rest pain, which is closely affiliated with a severe form of PAD. The patient may also experience pain throughout their feet and even in the heels especially when they are in the resting position with their legs at or above the level of their heart. In this position, the patient may also notice their feet changing from their normal color and becoming pale. Often, the pain dissipates when the individual sits or stands up, which allows blood flow to reach the feet once again. This change of positioning will also return the normal color to their feet as gravity enables the blood to move to a more distal location. Ischemic rest pain does not affect the calf muscles.

Copyright © Mometrix Media. You have been licensed one copy of this document for personal use only. Any other reproduction or redistribution is strictly prohibited. All rights reserved.
This content is provided for test preparation purposes only and does not imply an endorsement by Mometrix of any particular political, scientific, or religious point of view.

Helpfulness of Calculating the Acceleration Time

It can be helpful to calculate the acceleration time during an arterial study to discern if the patient's symptoms are due to inflow or outflow conditions. If an obstruction of the artery is present in the region of the blood vessel that is proximal to where the vascular technologist has the transducer, there will be a longer amount of time between the start of systole and the greatest peak velocity. On the other hand, the acceleration time will not be longer if the patient has a significant stenosis or occlusion in the region of the artery that is in a more distal location to where the artery is being interrogated. Notably, an example of inflow disease would be an aortoiliac stenosis because it refers to problems of blood traveling into the legs from the heart. An example of outflow disease would be a stenosis because blood is attempting to travel from the femoral artery to the rest of the lower extremity.

If the acceleration time of the CFA was calculated to be 145 msec, explain why this is considered to be an abnormal finding.

When evaluating the acceleration time of the CFA, it is considered to be abnormal if this number is greater than or equal to 133 msec. Because 145 msec is greater than 133 msec, the acceleration time of this particular patient is abnormal, and it correlates to significant disease of the iliac artery. To gain a better understanding of an abnormal finding, it is also important to study the appearance of the arterial waveform. The acceleration time is considered to be abnormal if there is a slow upslope from the beginning of systole to the maximum peak velocity. When there is a rapid upslope demonstrated from the beginning of systole to the maximum peak velocity, the acceleration time is considered to be normal.

Copyright © Mometrix Media. You have been licensed one copy of this document for personal use only. Any other reproduction or redistribution is strictly prohibited. All rights reserved.
This content is provided for test preparation purposes only and does not imply an endorsement by Mometrix of any particular political, scientific, or religious point of view.

Venous Peripheral Vasculature

Upper Extremity Veins

Superficial and Deep Veins

The deep venous system is a network of veins that acts as a conduit to return blood from the systemic circulatory system back to the heart. The deep veins usually have an artery that can be tracked parallel to the vein. The deep veins are often in a more internal location when compared to the superficial veins, which are found near the surface. The ulnar and radial veins are paired vessels (meaning there are two of them), are located near the ulnar artery and radial artery, and are considered deep veins. The axillary vein, brachial vein, and deep palmar venous arch are also part of the deep venous system. The cephalic and basilic veins are not joined by an artery with the same label and are not paired; instead, they are part of the superficial venous system. Note that the cephalic vein runs along the lateral portion of the arm, whereas the basilic vein is found on the medial aspect of the arm (remember the correct anatomical position).

Avoiding Confusion Using Terminology

The veins carry blood that has been depleted of oxygen back to the heart. Because of the direction that blood travels within the veins, it is helpful to use terminology that will help avoid any confusion in regard to which segment of the vessel is being examined or discussed. Often, the terms proximal and distal are used, but it can often be helpful when evaluating the veins of the upper extremities to use the terms cranial and caudal instead. Transverse imaging is 90 degrees (or perpendicular) to the vein's long axis. The longitudinal imaging plane is parallel to the long axis of the blood vessel.

Brachiocephalic Veins vs. the Brachiocephalic Artery

The venous system consists of bilateral brachiocephalic veins. The right and left brachiocephalic veins are also referred to as the right and left innominate veins, which allow the blood to flow from the internal jugular and subclavian veins on both sides of the body. Collectively, these vessels aid in returning blood that has been depleted of oxygen from regions superior to the heart back to the right atrium via the SVC when they merge. It is important to note that the arterial system varies, however, because there is only one brachiocephalic artery that stems from the aortic arch. This is also known as the innominate artery, and it supplies oxygenated blood to the right side of the neck, the head, as well as the right upper extremity. The innominate artery can supply these anatomical structures because it branches into the right carotid and subclavian arteries.

Lower Extremity Veins

Protocol and Sonographic Findings When Negative for a DVT

The venous system is a network of veins that returns blood that has been depleted of oxygen back to the right atrium of the heart. The vessel walls of veins and arteries consist of three separate layers, but the layers in veins tend to be thinner, which allows the vessel to be compressed during a venous duplex exam. A venous duplex exam is performed to diagnose the presence of a deep vein thrombosis (DVT). The protocol includes gray-scale, color, and spectral Doppler starting at the groin in the transverse plane compressing the veins with light pressure from the transducer. A vein that can be compressed wall to wall does not contain a clot (which can usually be seen with gray-scale and color Doppler). Nonobstructed veins above the knee should demonstrate spontaneous flow and phasicity with changes in respiration. Some labs also use augmentation to show that there isn't a clot between the calf and a more proximal location that is being scanned.

Copyright © Mometrix Media. You have been licensed one copy of this document for personal use only. Any other reproduction or redistribution is strictly prohibited. All rights reserved.
This content is provided for test preparation purposes only and does not imply an endorsement by Mometrix of any particular political, scientific, or religious point of view.

Improving Color Doppler Images with Persistence

Persistence is an averaging technique that will combine images from older frames with those of newer data. In gray-scale imaging, persistence can be used to smooth out an image or reduce the amount of noise that is present. Persistence is also found to be useful in color Doppler imaging, especially if the vessels to be visualized are deeper in the body (such as in cases of obese patients or edema), to identify vessels that contain slow-moving blood, or if there is an obstruction of a vessel. Smaller blood vessels can also be identified more readily than with methods that do not implement persistence. It is important to note that the temporal resolution is often decreased when persistence is applied to an image.

Difficulty Visualizing the Femoral Vein

During a venous duplex exam, the femoral vein is often difficult to visualize well in the distal thigh because it tends to run deeper in the lower third of the leg when compared to the mid and proximal thigh as it is approached from the popliteal region. The popliteal vein advances through an area known as the adductor hiatus (also referred to as Hunter's canal). This area contains an opening that allows the passage of the popliteal vein to course from the posterior portion of the knee to the anterior thigh. In the distal thigh, the vascular technologist may find it helpful to interrogate the distal femoral vein on the posterior surface instead of from a more medial or anterior approach.

Inguinal Ligament as a Landmark for Vascular Imaging

The femoral triangle is an important anatomical region that physicians use when the femoral vein or artery needs to be used as an access point. The femoral triangle is located at the anterior portion of the thigh, and the inguinal ligament marks the superior-most border of the femoral triangle. The inguinal ligament is a structure that separates the thigh from the wall of the abdominal cavity. The inguinal ligament may be palpated by physicians in patients who are thin when vascular access is necessary. Vascular technologists should use the inguinal ligament as a landmark to discern the external iliac artery from the common femoral artery (CFA) because this vessel becomes the CFA once it travels past and underneath it. The common femoral vein (CFV) is formed within the femoral triangle when the deep femoral vein (DFV) meets the superficial femoral vein (SFV). The CFV is found just medial to the CFA. The great saphenous vein (GSV) enters the CFV before it passes underneath the inguinal ligament, which then gives way to the vessel known as the external iliac vein.

Hunter's Canal

The area known as Hunter's canal is an important region located near the knee because it serves as a tunnel that allows the blood vessels of the thigh and lower leg to pass through the region of the popliteal fossa. For example, the femoral artery enters the posterior area of the knee to become the popliteal artery. The popliteal vein also passes through this region to become the femoral vein in the distal thigh. Often, the distal femoral vein cannot be seen due the depth of the vein in the area of Hunter's canal, so it may be necessary to scan from a more posterior approach. Another name for Hunter's canal is the adductor canal.

Popliteal Trifurcation

The area of the lower extremity known as the popliteal trifurcation is where the anterior tibial artery and the tibioperoneal trunk branch from the peroneal artery in the posterior region of the knee. This is an important area to evaluate because it is a common site for atherosclerosis to develop. The anterior tibial artery is the first artery to stem from the popliteal artery, and it courses along the anterior (front) of the lower leg to become the dorsalis pedis artery (DPA). The tibioperoneal trunk is the second arterial segment to divide from the peroneal artery. This trunk

Copyright © Mometrix Media. You have been licensed one copy of this document for personal use only. Any other reproduction or redistribution is strictly prohibited. All rights reserved.
This content is provided for test preparation purposes only and does not imply an endorsement by Mometrix of any particular political, scientific, or religious point of view.

bifurcates to form the peroneal artery, which supplies blood to the lateral region of the lower leg as well as the posterior tibial artery (PTA). The PTA runs along the medial side of the leg to carry blood to the foot.

Scenario

Spectral Doppler demonstrates continuous flow of the popliteal vein in a patient that presents with pain in the calf and associated swelling. The patient also describes a fullness in the popliteal fossa. Explain if this would likely be a positive or negative venous duplex study and what else the vascular technologist should evaluate for.

In a patient that presents with a fullness in the popliteal fossa and continuous flow of the popliteal vein when examined with spectral Doppler, the vascular technologist should also evaluate the popliteal fossa. The fullness behind the knee, pain, and swelling could be caused by a Baker's cyst. A Baker's cyst can create a fluid collection in the posteromedial portion of the knee joint, which could compress the popliteal vein to cause the continuous signal within. If a dedicated venous duplex exam was also performed, it would likely be negative for DVT because a ruptured Baker's cyst can cause pain and swelling of the calf.

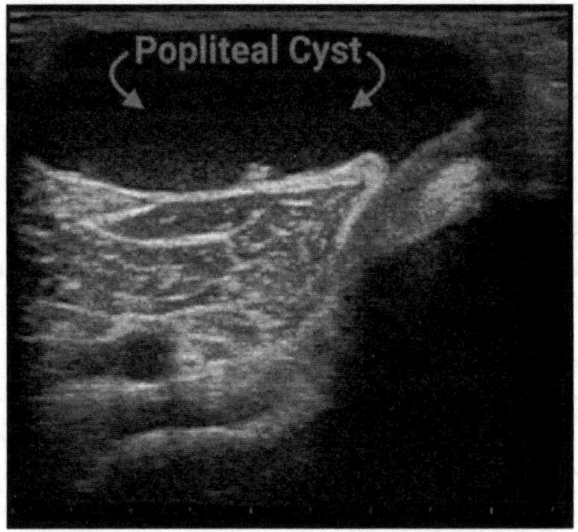

Popliteal Entrapment Syndrome

Popliteal entrapment syndrome is caused when the popliteal artery is compressed by the head of the gastrocnemius muscle, which, when contracted, decreases blood flow to the lower portion of the leg. This condition may be the result of a congenital anomaly of the gastrocnemius muscle, or it may develop as a result of athletic training and hypertrophy of the calf muscle (this can occur bilaterally). This condition typically arises in young men (often younger than the age of 30) who are athletes. If an active athlete describes symptoms of intermittent swelling, cramping, numbness, and aching during physical activity that disappear shortly after running, then the physician should consider popliteal entrapment syndrome even though this is a rare condition. When testing is performed, it should be done with and without muscle contraction for comparison, and if it is positive for entrapment a decrease of perfusion will be evident during contraction.

Great Saphenous Vein

The longest vein in the body is the great saphenous vein (GSV), which is found in the medial surface of the legs. There is a right and left GSV, and these vessels start on the top of the foot and ascend anteriorly to the medial malleoli while continuing to the saphenofemoral junction (SFJ). The SFJ is where the GSV finally merges with the common femoral vein (CFV) in the patient's proximal thigh. The GSV does contain valves, and more of these structures are located inferior to the knee. The GSV

Copyright © Mometrix Media. You have been licensed one copy of this document for personal use only. Any other reproduction or redistribution is strictly prohibited. All rights reserved.
This content is provided for test preparation purposes only and does not imply an endorsement by Mometrix of any particular political, scientific, or religious point of view.

can receive blood from the entire leg because of the various tributaries that drain blood into it. The GSV is known as a superficial vein not only because of its superficial location, but because there is not an artery associated with it. The GSV is often harvested for use as a graft during coronary artery bypass surgery.

Vein Mapping

Vein mapping is performed when the patient is scheduled for a coronary artery bypass graft or if a dialysis site is needed. Deep veins are not harvested as bypass vessels, so only those in the superficial system are examined. The great saphenous vein (GSV), which is the longest vein in the body, is often the first vessel to be interrogated; it is found in the medial portion of the leg and courses from the top of the foot to the groin. If the GSV is not suitable for a bypass graft, then the small saphenous vein (SSV) may be used instead. However, if neither saphenous vein can be used due to disease within, small size, or if it has already been removed, the vascular technologist should evaluate the superficial veins of the upper extremities. The cephalic vein, which is found in the lateral portion of the upper extremity, is the preferred vessel, but the basilic vein could also be used.

Gastrocnemius and Soleal Veins

In order to assist in the blood return from the lower extremities to the heart, the gastrocnemius and soleal muscles must act as a muscle pump (with the soleal sinuses acting as the main supply). The contractions in the calf and ankle region aid in blood return by forcing the blood that is in the veins to move toward the heart when walking or performing any motion that flexes the foot. It is important to note that the gastrocnemius and soleal veins can develop blood clots; these may be seen during lower venous duplex exams. There are typically multiple gastrocnemius veins found in the calf region that drain directly into the popliteal vein of the lower leg. These vessels contain functioning valves. Deep vein thromboses (DVTs) that develop in the soleal veins are believed to be responsible for a large percentage of pulmonary emboli. The soleal sinuses tend to drain into the peroneal and posterior tibial veins.

Importance of the Calf Muscle Pump

An important component of the lower extremities to preserve normal blood return to the heart is known as the calf muscle pump. This system is comprised of veins that serve as a storage receptacle for blood, calf muscles, and internal venous valves that are competent and able to ensure one-way blood flow. When a patient walks or flexes the foot, the muscles within the calf act as a pump that squeezes the veins as the muscles contract. The ejection fraction of this venous/skeletal pump should be greater than 60% to prevent venous insufficiency.

Veins, like arteries, have three separate layers that make up the wall of the blood vessels. The walls of veins are less muscular than those of arteries. The middle layer (adventitia media) of veins is the thinnest component. Because veins tend to be less muscular, they are less elastic than arteries. Veins dilate in patients with venous insufficiency due to the pooling of blood in the distal portions of the lower extremities. When blood starts to collect due to incompetent valves, venous stasis can occur and will also contribute to the dilation of calf veins. The rise of hydrostatic pressure can create an expansion of the veins as well.

Soleal and Gastrocnemius Veins

The calf muscles have two groups of veins that return blood to the heart, which have the same name as the muscles that make up the calf (soleal and gastrocnemius veins). It is important to note that these veins drain into separate deep vessels. The soleal vein returns blood into the peroneal and posterior tibial veins via 10 or more sinusoids. The two segments of the gastrocnemius vein exit

Copyright © Mometrix Media. You have been licensed one copy of this document for personal use only. Any other reproduction or redistribution is strictly prohibited. All rights reserved.
This content is provided for test preparation purposes only and does not imply an endorsement by Mometrix of any particular political, scientific, or religious point of view.

both heads of the gastrocnemius muscles and empty into the medial and lateral portions of popliteal vein. If a patient develops a DVT within the gastrocnemius vein, it is important during a venous duplex follow-up exam to determine if the blood clot has propagated into the popliteal vein, which is one of the larger deep veins. If the blood clot is only within one of the calf muscle veins, it is referred to as an isolated calf muscle thrombosis.

Ascending vs. Descending Venography Exams

Venograms require the use of contrast to be injected and X-ray equipment to take sequential images of the veins. These exams can be uncomfortable for patients and require extreme technical expertise to read and perform the exams. Ascending venography can be used in the upper and lower extremities, whereas descending venography is only performed of the lower extremities. During an ascending venogram, the physician will inject the contrast into either the basilic or cephalic vein for the upper extremities and into a vein on the top of the foot if the lower extremity is being examined. Ascending venography can determine if a DVT or varicosities are present, if the patient has had previous blood clots, and the presence of collateral vessels. A descending venogram requires injection of contrast via the common femoral vein to assess the function of the valves (venous incompetence) as well as assessing for reflux.

Perforating and Communicating Veins

Perforating veins (also referred to as perforators) can be thought of as the vessels that join the superficial venous system to the deep veins. In fact, the pathway of blood draining from the lower limbs passes through the superficial veins into the perforators and then moves into the deep venous system. These veins are typically located within the muscle and are associated with a perforating artery. These vessels contain valves to ensure one-way blood flow to help blood reach the deep system such as those in the thigh and lower leg. Notably, the perforators located in the foot move blood into the superficial system instead of the deep system. There are also vessels known as communicating veins, which allow blood to travel in the same venous systems, for example, from the superficial venous system to superficial veins or from the deep venous system to deep veins. These are typically very small (less than 2 mm) and cannot typically be seen during a venous duplex ultrasound.

Primary and Secondary Varicose Veins

Varicose veins appear as tortuous, enlarged veins that develop when these vessels become overdistended with blood and allow pooling within. Veins that work normally tend to allow the propagation of blood flow from the lower extremities to the heart. When valves no longer work properly, retrograde flow tends to cause enlargement of the veins. Primary varicose veins are diagnosed when only the superficial system is affected by valvular incompetence. Sometimes, this is due to the congenital absence of valves, which can cause an increase of the venous pressure that does not affect the deep veins. Secondary varicose veins, however, do involve the deep venous system. These circumstances could include a prior DVT, which in turn damages the valves to allow retrograde flow. Secondary varicose veins also involve the incompetence of the superficial valves as well.

Provide Guidance for Venous Ablation Procedures

Ultrasound Prior to Ablation

The role that ultrasound plays prior to an ablation is to diagnose which sections of the varicose veins demonstrate reflux. The depth of the vessels should also be noted to determine any necessary precautions that may need to be taken to prevent extensive tissue damage. The size of the vessel must be measured to help determine if ablation can take place. Vascular technologists can map how

Copyright © Mometrix Media. You have been licensed one copy of this document for personal use only. Any other reproduction or redistribution is strictly prohibited. All rights reserved.
This content is provided for test preparation purposes only and does not imply an endorsement by Mometrix of any particular political, scientific, or religious point of view.

the vein travels as well as document how far this blood vessel is from the GSV. Documentation should also include the distance from the vein of interest distally to the region of the knee.

Ultrasound During Ablation

The vascular technologist will assist during an ablation procedure by setting up the tray and collecting the necessary supplies. The patient should be placed on the table and prepped, and sterile drapes should be used. The role of ultrasound for guidance should be to image the site that will be used. Often, if the access site is the GSV, then just above or below the knee is where the catheter or laser fiber will be placed. The ankle or distal calf region will be the area of placement if the SSV is of interest. Ultrasound should be used to make sure that the tool is 2–3 cm from the saphenofemoral location. Care should be taken so the catheter is not in the femoral vein because this could create a DVT if the vein is damaged. Anesthesia should be given, and ultrasound can document the correct placement so the patient will not feel as much heat and to prevent burns of the skin. Once the procedure is over, the catheter or laser fiber is taken out.

Radiofrequency Ablation vs. Endovenous Laser Ablation

When the clinical management of varicose veins is not successful, venous ablation is a treatment option. When patients have an incompetent GSV or SSV, varicose veins are often the result and venous ablation has been successful to ease painful symptoms. There is little difference between the types of venous ablation. Radiofrequency ablation is one type of treatment option that uses an electrode to impart radiofrequency energy on the wall of the veins in order to create closure of the vein as the heat makes the collagen within the vessel contract. This technique tends to create less postprocedure pain and bruising. Endovenous laser ablation is a venous ablation technique that enables users a more controlled use of heat due to the use of a tiny optic laser that closes the vein due to the contraction of the wall. This is the preferred method if small clots are present or if the vein has a larger diameter.

Color Doppler Exam and Postablation Workups

A vascular technologist may be required to perform a color Doppler exam of the lower extremity immediately afterward as part of the postablation workup to confirm that the GSV has been thrombosed accordingly, which will be confirmed if there is not color flow within the GSV in the region of the SFJ. The vascular technologist should also check the superficial epigastric branch in addition to the femoral vein to make sure that these vessels are patent and to evaluate for possible extension of the superficial venous thrombosis into the deep venous system.

Effect of Breathing on Blood Flow

When a spectral analysis of blood flow of the legs is performed in a patient that has patent veins, the signal will demonstrate phasic flow when the patient is breathing. In the lower extremities, the signal decreases upon inhalation and increases when the patient exhales. When the patient inhales, there is increased intra-abdominal pressure, which, in turn, lessens the flow from the legs. Upon exhalation, there is decreased intra-abdominal pressure, which enables the blood flow from the legs to increase. Vascular technologists should be aware that the opposite is true when assessing the upper extremities because the signal increases with inhalation and decreases when the patient exhales. When the Valsalva maneuver is performed, pressure in the thoracic and abdominal cavities rises, which creates a cessation of flow to the heart that interrupts all blood flow in the body.

Venous Insufficiency

Oxygenated blood is carried away from the heart in arteries, whereas blood that has been depleted of oxygen is returned to the heart in blood vessels known as veins. Veins have internal structures known as valves that stem from the same tissue that makes up the innermost layer of the wall of the

Copyright © Mometrix Media. You have been licensed one copy of this document for personal use only. Any other reproduction or redistribution is strictly prohibited. All rights reserved.
This content is provided for test preparation purposes only and does not imply an endorsement by Mometrix of any particular political, scientific, or religious point of view.

vein and assist in moving the blood toward the heart. These valves, when working correctly, also prevent blood flow from traveling in the wrong direction. Incompetent valves enable the blood to flow backward (as well as in a normal antegrade direction). This reflux precipitates pooling of blood in the legs, which leads to what is known as chronic venous insufficiency (CVI). Pressure within the vessels becomes increased, and fluid and blood may seep into the surrounding tissue, which is why people with CVI often have a brown color in their limbs. Up to 75% of ulcers that develop in the lower extremity are due to CVI.

Common Ultrasound Characteristics of a DVT

The common ultrasound appearance of a deep vein thrombosis (DVT) is a vein that is dilated. During a venous duplex ultrasound, the vascular technologist will not be able to compress the vein wall to wall. The vascular technologist may notice during the exam that the thrombus does not appear to be completely attached to the wall of the blood vessel (this may be more noticeable in the sagittal plane when scanning the distal portion of the thrombus because motion may be discerned). An acute DVT may appear more hypoechoic than a chronic clot, which tends to be more echogenic. Often with chronic changes, synechiae will be apparent within the affected vessel(s), which represent the lysis and contraction of the clot. The arrow in this ultrasound image demonstrates a thrombus that is present in the left CFV. Chronic clots may also demonstrate recanalized and/or collateral vessels.

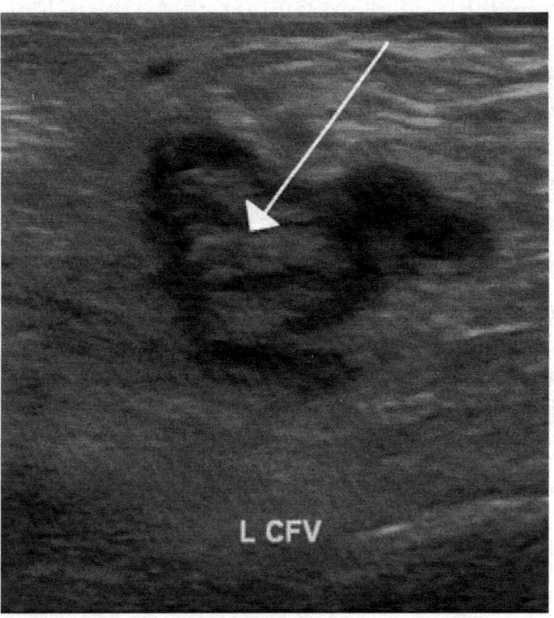

Common Ultrasound Characteristics of a DVT

If a patient develops an acute DVT, the main clinical concern is a pulmonary embolism (PE). A PE occurs when part of the thrombus, or in some cases the entire clot, breaks off and travels within the circulatory system and becomes lodged in one of the pulmonary arteries, which can be fatal. In cases that are not fatal, damage to the lungs or other organs can occur because the amount of oxygenated blood is reduced due to the obstruction. Patients that have a PE will often present with shortness of breath or chest pain. Typically, a PE is the result of a DVT in the lower extremities. The symptoms of a DVT in the extremities often include pain, swelling, warmth, and redness. DVTs can occur when an individual does not move for long periods of time such as after long flights or even after surgery. Some patients develop them because of hormone-related medicines such as birth control. Other individuals have a genetic predisposition to blood clots.

Copyright © Mometrix Media. You have been licensed one copy of this document for personal use only. Any other reproduction or redistribution is strictly prohibited. All rights reserved.
This content is provided for test preparation purposes only and does not imply an endorsement by Mometrix of any particular political, scientific, or religious point of view.

CVI Common for Those with a Previous DVT

In patients that have had a previous DVT, the most common complication is chronic venous insufficiency ([CVI] a pulmonary embolism is the most severe life-threatening complication). This is also referred to as post-thrombotic syndrome when venous insufficiency occurs because of a blood clot. If a DVT forms and propagates, it can cause permanent distension of the walls of the veins while creating scar tissue within the blood vessel itself. This scar tissue can extend to the internal valves, which creates the inability to ensure one-way blood flow (valvular incompetence). When the direction of blood flow within the veins no longer only propagates toward the heart, the blood can pool within the vessels, which increases the amount of venous pressure. The calf and ankle area often become edematous because of blood, fluids, and fibrinogen escaping into the adjacent tissues because of the rise in venous pressure.

Source of Thrombosis When a Patient Experiences a PE

A PE typically derives from a DVT of the lower extremities. Although not all clinicians agree about the treatment and management of DVTs when found in the lower leg, the most common source of thrombosis, which causes deadly PE, is the soleal vein. This occurrence takes place because the soleal muscle only functions in the area of the ankle (unlike the gastrocnemius muscle, which functions throughout the entire lower leg). When individuals are not able to move either because of an injury or an inability to walk, or if they are on a long car ride or flight, the soleal vein can become sluggish and not drain normally because it is not contracting. The soleal veins drain into the peroneal and posterior tibial veins.

Development of Venous Ulcers

Ulcers are open wounds or sores that develop when there is an interruption of circulation to parts of the body. Ulcers may be the result of venous and/or arterial disease such as CVI or PAD. Venous ulcers materialize when there is valvular incompetency and the blood pools in the lower leg and ankle area. Edema and venous hypertension are responsible for the typical location of these venous ulcers because they are found most of the time in the region known as the gaiter zone, which is the area just above the medial and lateral malleoli. In the area of the medial malleolus, several important perforators are found, which is why the tissue breakdown is evident here. Ulcers of venous origin in this area do not typically hurt as much as those that stem from arterial disease. However, these ulcers do tend to ooze, and if the ulcers are characterized as "wet," they are associated as venous stasis ulcers, which have a high correlation with venous insufficiency.

Comparing the Phasicity of Both Sides

A vascular technologist should perform a complete venous duplex exam on the affected side to rule out a DVT for swelling, even if the exam is negative for a DVT from the CFV distally. However, the protocol for a unilateral exam should include a spectral Doppler waveform of the contralateral side (CFV) to compare phasicity signals. The vascular technologist should perform this comparison while scanning in the long axis with the patient in the exact same position that the affected side was scanned. If there is a discrepancy noted with phasicity or if the waveform appears continuous, which means it isn't affected at all during respiration, then it is important to look for an obstruction in a more proximal location. Some labs may require both external iliac veins to also be interrogated to compare respiratory phasicity. If a patient has an obstructive thrombosis of the iliofemoral veins, it can cause pallor and excessive swelling; this is a condition referred to as phlegmasia alba dolens.

Managing CVI

It is important to diagnose and manage CVI as quickly as possible before tissues break down and ulcers develop. Patients need to understand the importance of proper nutrition, exercise, and

Copyright © Mometrix Media. You have been licensed one copy of this document for personal use only. Any other reproduction or redistribution is strictly prohibited. All rights reserved.
This content is provided for test preparation purposes only and does not imply an endorsement by Mometrix of any particular political, scientific, or religious point of view.

taking steps to care for their skin. When skin infections are present, antibiotics may need to be prescribed. Individuals with CVI must avoid sitting for extended periods to prevent the blood from pooling in the lower legs. Also, the patient should try to rest with their feet up after it is necessary to be on their feet. Physicians may prescribe compression stockings as well. If ulcers are already present, medicated (Unna) boots and dressings may be the first treatment step. If these are not effective, the patient may need to be treated with several sessions of hyperbaric oxygen therapy.

Venous Aneurysm

A venous aneurysm is a dilation of a vein that is 1.5 times larger than the adjacent segments of the same vessel. Venous aneurysms are not very common, but when seen they may affect men or women of any age. They typically involve the veins of the legs and, more specifically, the popliteal vein, but they may occur in the jugular and upper extremities as well. Venous aneurysms may include complications such as blood clots or emboli, especially those that are diagnosed in the deep veins. Most individuals with a venous aneurysm complain of pain, swelling, and a palpable mass if the deep system is involved. If present in the groin region, they may be difficult to diagnose correctly without imaging because the symptoms are similar to those of a hernia. Surgery is often the course of action when a venous aneurysm is found.

Virchow's Triad

In patients that have acquired a DVT, at least one of three risk factors must have taken place. Collectively, these circumstances are known as Virchow's triad. The first possible component is trauma, which could include something as simple as the placement of an IV or a blood draw that injures the wall of the vein. The second risk factor is stasis, which occurs when blood moves through the body more slowly than normal. Stasis can occur when a patient is bedridden or travels long distances while sitting, such as a long plane ride. Any time the blood starts to circulate at a slower pace or stop, a DVT is more likely to occur. The third component is hypercoagulability, which can be inherited, as is the case of factor V Leiden, acquired in individuals with cancer or women who use certain birth control methods, such as pills, rings, or patches.

Ultrasound and Clinical Findings

Patients that present to the vascular lab with a positive diagnosis of an acute DVT often complain of pain, swelling, and redness of the affected extremity. They may also complain of the extremity being warm to the touch. In situations in which the blood clot has traveled to the lungs, the patient may also explain symptoms of crushing chest pain and shortness of breath. Ultrasound findings of an acute DVT include the inability to completely compress the lumen of the affected vein(s). Gray-scale imaging will also demonstrate homogenous, low-level filling defects inside the vein that do not appear to adhere to the walls. Often, veins that are thrombosed will appear larger than normal. Color Doppler will not demonstrate complete filling of the vessel.

Treatment Options for Risk of Losing a Leg

In the majority of patients that have been diagnosed with a DVT, the patient is able to undergo anticoagulation therapy in order to treat the blood clot. Although these blood thinners do not dissolve the clot, their purpose is to prevent the clot from breaking off or becoming bigger. Thrombolytics may be necessary for some patients that are not responding well to the current blood thinner or who have developed pulmonary emboli. However, in some individuals the blood clot may be so extensive that even thrombolytic drugs won't work, especially if the iliofemoral portions are involved. In these cases, an iliofemoral venous thrombectomy may be the patient's best option to reduce complications such as the need to amputate the extremity, especially if it is treated early. New technology for a venous thrombectomy have improved the outcomes for the patient

Copyright © Mometrix Media. You have been licensed one copy of this document for personal use only. Any other reproduction or redistribution is strictly prohibited. All rights reserved.
This content is provided for test preparation purposes only and does not imply an endorsement by Mometrix of any particular political, scientific, or religious point of view.

with fewer complications and significantly higher postprocedure patency rates without compromising valvular activity.

Copyright © Mometrix Media. You have been licensed one copy of this document for personal use only. Any other reproduction or redistribution is strictly prohibited. All rights reserved.
This content is provided for test preparation purposes only and does not imply an endorsement by Mometrix of any particular political, scientific, or religious point of view.

Extracranial Cerebral Vasculature and Other Procedures

NONIMAGING PHYSIOLOGIC EXAM VS. DUPLEX ULTRASOUND STUDY

A nonimaging physiologic exam is performed to test at least one region of the extremities to determine the presence of disease as well as the significance. Physiologic exams are considered to be indirect studies, but the vascular technologist should always examine the right and left sides so comparisons can be made. Physiologic exams should include the ankle-brachial indices (ABIs) to be calculated by obtaining continuous-wave or pulse volume recordings at the wrist or ankle level. Duplex ultrasound studies involve the use of color and spectral Doppler interrogation and allow for direct evaluation of disease within a specific section of the artery. Duplex ultrasound studies should also be performed bilaterally in order to offer a comparison for a more detailed diagnosis.

IMPORTANCE OF REST PRIOR TO EXAM

When performing physiologic arterial exams, it may be taxing for the patient to make his or her way back to the ultrasound lab, so it is important to have the patient rest before starting the exam. By allowing the patient to rest for at least five minutes (even more time is better) before the vascular technologist starts the exam, this should provide sufficient time for the blood flow to return to normal before the start of the exam. If this rest time is not afforded to the patient, incorrect testing results could be made. While the vascular technologist is explaining the exam to the patient, the patient should be instructed to lie on his or her back and place the arms down by their sides. The head of the bed can be raised slightly in order to allow the patient to rest comfortably. It is important to be aware of the temperature of the room as well as keeping the patient covered if he or she is cold.

PHOTOPLETHYSMOGRAPHY

Photoplethysmography (PPG) is often used to determine if arterial disease is present in the digits (fingers and toes) by sending an infrared light into the prominent tissue of the finger so the light that is reflected will represent the amount of cutaneous blood flow. Prior to the exam, it is important that the vascular technologist determine if the patient is anxious about the exam because the results can be skewed if this is the case because stress can induce a narrowing of the arteries and affect blood pressure. Answering all questions that the patient may have about the test so he or she knows what to expect should alleviate the amount of nervousness that is felt. It is important that the vascular technologist also asks if the patient is cold because vasoconstriction will alter the effectiveness of the test. Yet another factor that impacts the arteries to cause vasoconstriction is smoking, so it is important to find out if the patient has smoked recently.

EVALUATING FINGERS WITH PLETHYSMOGRAPHY

If a physician is trying to rule out Raynaud's phenomenon, the vascular technologist may need to examine the patient's fingers with and without cold stress. The technique first evaluates the patient without cold stress while keeping the patient warm. In order to eliminate the possibility of disease in the proximal vessels, the sonographer should obtain bilateral brachial artery pressures as well as pressures of the forearm. Recall that the ulnar and radial arteries deliver oxygenated blood to the hand, so it is necessary to also evaluate the palmar arch. The fingertips of the digits that are of concern will be evaluated by waveform and pressure plethysmography. For the cold stress, the patient's hands will be placed in ice water until it becomes unbearable or for a maximum of three minutes. It is important to note any changes in skin color or symptoms that the patient has as well as how long the patient's hands were immersed in the ice water. Although the exam is performed bilaterally, if one side is of greater concern, that side should be examined first. The same method is used immediately after wiping off the water and is repeated again five minutes later.

Copyright © Mometrix Media. You have been licensed one copy of this document for personal use only. Any other reproduction or redistribution is strictly prohibited. All rights reserved.
This content is provided for test preparation purposes only and does not imply an endorsement by Mometrix of any particular political, scientific, or religious point of view.

Using Cold Stress

Cold stress PPG testing is an important method to perform if true vasospasm is suspected in an individual because the blood flow to the digits can be normal when the patient is tested without cold stress. With this evaluation, the waveforms and pressures should be performed at room temperature with the patient at a comfortable temperature. Cold stress testing requires the patient to place their hands in ice water for three minutes or until it becomes unbearable. It is considered abnormal if the patient's waveforms do not return to the levels of those that were seen before cold stress was applied by the five-minute mark. Normally, the amplitude of the waveform is hardly impacted by the ice water, but when the patient experiences vasospasm, the peaks demonstrate a rounded appearance.

Obtaining Toe Pressures

The method used to obtain toe pressures is usually done in conjunction with a physiologic arterial exam of the lower extremities. However, if ordered separately, it is important to eliminate the possibility of disease in the proximal arteries, so bilateral ABIs will be calculated first. Either volume or photoplethysmographic waveforms are obtained from the great toes as well as any other toes that are of concern. Some labs use continuous-wave Doppler for the pressures with volume or photo techniques, but this can be technically challenging because it can be difficult to stay on the tiny digital arteries. The cuff will be placed at the base of the great toe, and the photocell is applied to the undersurface of the distal portion of the same digit. The sonographer will inflate the cuff at the same time that the arterial pulses are being recorded. Once the cuff is 20–30 mmHg more than the highest ankle pressure systolic reading, the pulsation should stop, which prompts the technologist to deflate the cuff. When the pulse appears again in the PPG tracing, the toe pressure is documented.

Normal Limits of Fingers and Toes

Normal PPG studies that are performed of the fingers and toes are considered to be within normal limits if the waveform demonstrates a sharp upstroke at the same time of peak systole. There should also be a downstroke that is lengthy with a dicrotic notch visualized about halfway through the downstroke. It is important to note that the waveforms of the toes tend to have a smaller amplitude when compared to the amplitude of the fingers. Abnormal qualities include a slow upstroke, with a dicrotic notch appearing in a high location of the downstroke (instead of halfway down). If an occlusion is present proximally to the most distal portion of the digit, the waveform will tend to have a more rounded appearance of the peak with a slow upstroke. Raynaud's phenomenon often demonstrates a PPG waveform that has a peaked pulse.

Advantages and Disadvantages of PPG

PPG uses a photocell that is placed slightly above the medial malleolus while the patient is sitting with his or her legs hanging off the table. This modality is a noninvasive test that can be used to evaluate venous and arterial blood flow. The venous PPG will use the DC mode because it detects blood that is moving more slowly. PPG is used to determine if venous insufficiency is present and its significance. The photocell should not be used in areas of skin that are broken or ulcerated, and it should not be placed over a varicose vein because doing so can provide false data. Another problem that the vascular technologist may encounter is that unusually thick skin may hinder the propagation of the infrared light into the subcutaneous tissue.

Dorsiflexion Maneuver During a PPG Study

While the patient sits upright with his or her legs hanging off the table, the vascular technologist will ask the patient to dorsiflex the foot. During these studies with various maneuvers, the vascular

Copyright © Mometrix Media. You have been licensed one copy of this document for personal use only. Any other reproduction or redistribution is strictly prohibited. All rights reserved.
This content is provided for test preparation purposes only and does not imply an endorsement by Mometrix of any particular political, scientific, or religious point of view.

technologist may have to demonstrate the action for the patient or give very specific instructions. The patient should perform an exaggerated dorsiflexion 5 to 10 times so the blood empties from the veins. In some cases, the individual may not be able to dorsiflex the foot well enough, so the sonographer can squeeze the calf for them. If manual compression is necessary on one side, the vascular technologist must perform this for the patent bilaterally in order to obtain comparable results. The venous refill time is obtained after completing the dorsiflexion exercises.

Air Plethysmography

Air plethysmography is also referred to as volume plethysmography. This modality can be used for venous and arterial testing. Venous applications are used to determine if CVI is present by determining the venous filling index, the ejection fraction, and the residual volume fraction while evaluating the patient in various positions and movements. This study is important to determine the filling of the veins as well as the depletion of the venous blood. The exam is performed after the application of a cuff that encircles the calf region first with the patient supine. The patient is then instructed to stand quickly for a couple of more measurements/movements and then will return to the supine position to deplete the blood from the veins once again.

Venous Filling Index

During an air plethysmography exam, once the vascular technologist determines the zero venous volume, the sonographer will ask the patient to stand up quickly from the supine position. The patient's test leg should be non-weight-bearing. Gravity will enable the blood to fill the veins of the lower leg once again. Then, the venous filling index (VFI) can be calculated to determine how fast the veins refill. The VFI is calculated using the following formula:

$$\text{VFI} = \frac{90\% \text{ venous volume}}{90\% \text{ venous filling time}}$$

A VFI of less than or equal to 2 is considered normal. If the VFI falls in the 2–10 range, it suggests that a minor to moderate reflux is present. If the VFI is greater than 10, then it is assumed that the patient has severe reflux.

Normal Ejection Fraction

When performing an air plethysmography study, it is considered normal if the ejection fraction (EF) is greater than 60%. After the venous filling index is found after the patient quickly stands from the supine position, the patient will stand on both feet and will be asked to exercise in order to stimulate the calf-muscle pump. This can be performed by asking the patient to perform one calf raise by having the patient stand on their tiptoes to the best of their ability. The EF is calculated with the following formula:

$$\text{EF} = \frac{\text{EV}}{\text{VV}} \times 100$$

where EV is the ejection volume and VV is the venous volume.

Residual Volume Fraction

When performing an air plethysmography study, the residual volume fraction (RVF) is one of the parameters that is calculated. A study is considered to be normal when the RVF is calculated to be less than 35%. The RVF is calculated after the EF (in which the patient performs 1 calf raise), and the vascular technologist will ask the patient to perform 10 more calf raises. This value determines

Copyright © Mometrix Media. You have been licensed one copy of this document for personal use only. Any other reproduction or redistribution is strictly prohibited. All rights reserved.
This content is provided for test preparation purposes only and does not imply an endorsement by Mometrix of any particular political, scientific, or religious point of view.

how much blood remains in the veins after having the patient perform this maneuver. The RVF is the ratio of the residual volume to the venous volume:

$$\mathrm{RVF} = \frac{\mathrm{RV}}{\mathrm{VV}}$$

Venous Refill Time

If the results of the venous refill time (VRT) is greater than or equal to 20 seconds, then the PPG study is determined to be within normal limits. If the VRT is less than 20 seconds, the exam is considered abnormal. If this is the case, the sonographer would continue the exam by wrapping a tourniquet around the patient's distal thigh region and the patient is instructed to dorsiflex his or her foot 5 to 10 times. The VRT is obtained once again, and if it is greater than 20 seconds then it is assumed that reflux is present in the GSV. The sonographer should continue the exam by applying the tourniquet just below the knee and asking the patient to dorsiflex the foot 5 to 10 times and repeat the tracings. At this point, it can be discerned that if the VRT is greater than 20 seconds with the tourniquet in place inferior to the knee that reflux is present in the SSV. It is suggested that incompetence of the deep system is present when a VRT of less than 20 seconds is found with and without the use of the tourniquet.

Sites for an AVF in the Upper Extremity

The radial artery and cephalic vein are common sites for an arteriovenous fistula (AVF) in the upper extremity because the forearm is favored over the use of the upper arm whenever possible. Typically, the nondominant forearm is used, and if it fails the dominant forearm is still the preferred access site over the upper arm, but in either case the cephalic vein will serve as the draining vein and will become distended for hemodialysis access. In contrast to an anastomosis created in the upper arm, when a hemodialysis access of the forearm is used, it is in a more superficial location than those of the upper arm, and this typically equates to less discomfort for the patient because it is easier to cannulate when the patient undergoes dialysis. Also, if the forearm access sites become thrombosed and fail, it is still possible to create a new access site more proximally, whereas the reverse situation does not typically work. If an access site in the upper arm is created first and fails, it is not likely that a forearm or more distal access site will be able to be used on the same arm.

Compartment Syndrome

Compartment syndrome is usually a diagnosis that is made clinically after an injury to the arms, legs, or less often the abdomen, and pressures within the compartment may be requested. The patient often presents with pain, swelling, muscle weakness, and numbness, and for cases that are more advanced it may be difficult to establish pulses in the extremity because they have become weakened or are not present. These symptoms are created due to bleeding that is associated with a great deal of swelling that occurs in the osteofascial compartments of the affected extremity. When this type of swelling develops, extrinsic compression reduces the blood flow so it can no longer reach the nerves or tissues and the muscle is at an increased risk of dying. Whether the case is acute or chronic, treatment includes a procedure called a fasciotomy, in which the contents of the compartment are cut open to allow for the swelling to dissipate.

Raynaud's Phenomenon

Raynaud's phenomenon can affect the fingers or toes when the blood supply to these regions is obstructed. There are two types of Raynaud's phenomenon, with the first being known as primary or idiopathic, which occurs intermittently in generally healthy patients. This stems from vasospasms within the hand and feet that supply oxygenated blood to the digits. This form is

Copyright © Mometrix Media. You have been licensed one copy of this document for personal use only. Any other reproduction or redistribution is strictly prohibited. All rights reserved.
This content is provided for test preparation purposes only and does not imply an endorsement by Mometrix of any particular political, scientific, or religious point of view.

believed to be hereditary and is common in young women especially when exposed to cold temperatures. Primary Raynaud's usually presents as discoloration of the digits bilaterally but with little to no pain. The prognosis tends to be positive for these individuals. Secondary Raynaud's is also known as obstructive Raynaud's and is the result of other underlying medical conditions such as autoimmune diseases or arthritis. Unlike the primary form of this disease, the ischemia always exists, and patients may have excruciating pain, numbness, and tingling due to an arterial obstruction that is constant even though the arterioles constrict normally.

Blue Toe Syndrome

If a patient presents to the emergency department or physician's office with a blue toe(s), the provider should consider blue toe syndrome. This condition will cause the toes to have a cyanotic appearance. This bluish/purplish discoloration is caused when small blood vessels are blocked by some sort of emboli. Mechanical obstruction can be caused when a thrombus breaks off, and the emboli become lodged in the tiny distal arteries of the toes. These emboli are primarily the result of atherosclerosis and are the main concern when a peripheral aneurysm is present in one of the arteries. These emboli could also be caused from gases or liquids such as contrast that was injected during an angiographic exam or anticoagulant treatment. Collateral arterial channels may form, which will alleviate the ischemia and discoloration of the affected digits.

Baker's Cyst

Synovial fluid is found in joint capsules, and it aids in the reduction of friction when an individual uses his or her limbs. If there is too much synovial fluid in the posterior knee, it is referred to as a Baker's cyst. This fluid collection will appear as a well-defined cystic component in the posterior and/or medial region within the popliteal fossa. Sometimes the patient may complain of a fullness behind their knee as well as pain, but often a Baker's cyst is an incidental finding without any symptoms. These fluid collections can occur because of an injury or because of inflammation associated with arthritis. These cysts may rupture, which occurs more often in patients who have osteoarthritis, gout, or in the elderly. During an ultrasound exam, a Baker's cyst that has ruptured will have a point as the fluid moves distally between the gastrocnemius and soleus muscles. The neck of this structure will be found between the semimembranosus tendon and the medial head of the gastrocnemius muscle.

Factors of Hemodynamically Stenosis

A stenotic lesion often turns into a hemodynamically stenosis when the diameter of the artery is reduced by half of the total for that vessel. The resulting area of the vessel would be 25% of the original cross section. A hemodynamically significant stenosis not only reduces the volume of blood flow, but also the pressure of the blood flowing. Other factors that influence if it will be a hemodynamically significant stenosis is how long the lesion is, the extensiveness of the stenosis, the shape that is formed from the lesion, the amount or presence of resistance that exists distal to the stenosis in the peripheral system, the texture of the surface of the arterial wall, and whether collateral channels are open for blood to pass through them.

Determining the Location of Collateral Channels

Collateral channels develop in arteries so that blood can bypass the region that is totally occluded or shows significant stenosis to reach the more distal regions. It can be helpful to perform Doppler segmental pressures when complete occlusion of an artery is present to help identify the level at which the blockage has occurred. In cases of a significant stenosis or complete occlusion, collateral channels will often materialize, which will still allow for a normal amount of blood flow when the patient is resting. When a blockage has occurred, the blood flow patterns in collaterals that are near

Copyright © Mometrix Media. You have been licensed one copy of this document for personal use only. Any other reproduction or redistribution is strictly prohibited. All rights reserved.
This content is provided for test preparation purposes only and does not imply an endorsement by Mometrix of any particular political, scientific, or religious point of view.

or at a more distant position could demonstrate increased velocities with a more pulsatile waveform and increased total volume of blood.

Effect of Hemodynamically Significant Stenosis

Laminar flow is the type of flow that is exhibited in patent blood vessels. If a clinician listens to the blood moving through a vessel with laminar flow, it will not be concerning. This flow is layered and smooth, and it travels parallel along the length of the vessel. If the diameter of the artery decreases by 50%, then it is assumed that the cross-sectional area has been decreased by 75% in the presence of a hemodynamically significant stenosis. When the diameter of the artery has been affected, the velocity of the blood flow will increase. If a provider hears an abnormal sound when listening with a stethoscope, this is known as a bruit. A bruit is caused by blood flow that is abnormally turbulent, but it may not be heard when a total occlusion or significant stenosis is present.

Spectral Broadening

A spectral Doppler waveform represents all of the velocities found in a sample of a blood within a particular vessel. Two types of flow can be ascertained in the sample. The first is normal, or laminar, flow, in which the spectral window is clear and the red blood cells are traveling at almost the same velocities. The second type of flow is turbulent flow, which shows movement that is disorganized because the blood is traveling at different speeds and various directions. Instead of a clear spectral window as seen in laminar flow, it appears to be filled in, which represents spectral broadening. Spectral broadening is a display of a broad range of Doppler shifts that are apparent within the sample of blood flow taken in a vessel. This may happen due to a stenotic or tortuous vessel.

Flow Patterns in Arteries with a Significant Stenosis

An artery that exhibits a significant stenosis typically presents predictable flow patterns that vascular technologists are familiar with when performing ultrasound exams. In the area of the artery proximal to the stenotic lesion, it is common to see diminished blood flow velocities that may or may not be moving chaotically. As the blood travels through the area of the artery that is narrowed, increased velocities will be noted. Normal flow now becomes disorganized due to the formation of eddy currents. In the segment of the artery distal to the stenosis, turbulence is commonly present. As the artery becomes wider, flow separation takes place at the arterial walls. Bidirectional blood flow is common in the area of poststenotic turbulence, but the velocity will be less than what was measured in the constricted portion of the artery.

Various Sounds Present in Arteries and Veins

Vascular technologists will typically be able to discern the various sounds that are present in arteries and veins. An arterial Doppler of the upper and lower extremities will show a pulsatile, high-frequency signal. A significant stenosis may be heard as an even higher pitched sound than a normal artery because the blood that is moving through the constricted lumen has increased velocities. Vascular technologists will also be able to tell when the transducer is placed in a more proximal and distal location to the segment of the artery that is stenotic. Recall that audible venous sounds will change with respiration and are usually considered to be of low frequency.

Appearance of Adequate Blood Flow Volume at Rest

When a patient is resting, there are various reasons why the volume of blood flow seems adequate even when there is a hemodynamically significant stenosis present. The first reason is that when a patient is resting, the amount of peripheral resistance will be less than that if the patient is active. Vasodilation, or a widening of the arteries, will allow more blood to pass through a vessel. However, if a person is exercising, the elevation of the pulse will create arterial constriction so the blood feeds

Copyright © Mometrix Media. You have been licensed one copy of this document for personal use only. Any other reproduction or redistribution is strictly prohibited. All rights reserved.
This content is provided for test preparation purposes only and does not imply an endorsement by Mometrix of any particular political, scientific, or religious point of view.

the muscles with oxygenated blood. Another reason for an apparent normal volume of flow when the patient has a hemodynamically significant stenosis is the formation of collateral channels, which enables the blood to flow around the part of the artery that is stenosed.

Appearance of Spectral Waveform

Any time a vascular technologist believes that a patient has a hemodynamically significant stenosis or occlusion of a peripheral artery, it is especially important to make sure that the Doppler parameters are set correctly. Of course, gray-scale, color, and spectral Doppler will be used to complete the ultrasound exam. If a patient has a hemodynamically significant stenosis of the leg, the waveform distal to the diseased artery likely demonstrates poststenotic turbulence and bidirectional flow may be seen as the blood is leaving the area of the blood vessel that is narrowed. Monophasic waveforms may also be present instead of the normal triphasic signals because the blood flow is not reversed. Some of the energy is lost because of the lesion, so there will be reduced peak velocities with the loss of the dicrotic notch.

Primary and Secondary Hypertension

Hypertension can be placed in one of two categories: primary or secondary. Primary hypertension (also referred to as essential hypertension) is the category in which a large percentage of the population falls into (95%). There appears to be no single, definitive cause of primary hypertension; rather, there is a combination of factors such as insulin resistance, aging, being overweight, poor nutrition, not getting enough (or any) exercise, a long-term considerable amount of alcohol consumption, and genetics. Secondary hypertension is known as renovascular hypertension. This type of high blood pressure is caused by a coexisting disorder that is already affecting the heart, arteries, kidneys, or endocrine system, or it is even caused by drug abuse. Although a small percentage of patients have this type of hypertension, it is usually due to the development of atherosclerosis and is found in patients that are older than 50.

Superior Thyroid Artery

The superior thyroid artery is a blood vessel that, as the name implies, is responsible for carrying oxygenated blood to the thyroid gland. The thyroid gland is a butterfly-shaped gland situated at the base of the neck near the midline. Its location explains why the direction of blood flow in the superior thyroid arterial branch moves in the opposite direction when compared to normal carotid arteries as it is moving inferior to the bottom of the neck. Vascular technologists can typically see the superior thyroid artery when performing a carotid duplex study because it is the first of eight branches of the external carotid artery (ECA). On occasion, the superior thyroid artery may arise from the distal segment of the CCA. The superior thyroid artery has several arterial branches to supply neighboring tissues.

Brain's Anterior Circulation vs. Posterior Circulation

The brain requires a constant supply of oxygenated blood in order to function, which demands blood from two sources. These two sources are intracranial in location but receive their blood from extracranial blood vessels. The anterior system supplies blood to the ophthalmic artery as well as the cerebrum from the ICAs. The anterior cerebral arteries (ACAs) and middle cerebral arteries (MCAs) arise from the ICA and create a vascular channel that has low resistance because of the constant supply of blood that is required. These vessels help establish the circle of Willis. The posterior circulatory system supplies the occipital lobe, cerebellum, and brain stem, which are all located in the posterior region of the cranium. Recall that the bilateral vertebral arteries join to form the basilar artery (known as the vertebrobasilar system), which gives rise to the posterior cerebral arteries (PCAs) to help establish the circle of Willis.

Copyright © Mometrix Media. You have been licensed one copy of this document for personal use only. Any other reproduction or redistribution is strictly prohibited. All rights reserved.
This content is provided for test preparation purposes only and does not imply an endorsement by Mometrix of any particular political, scientific, or religious point of view.

Circle of Willis

At the base of the brain, there is a network of vessels that is an anastomosis between the anterior and posterior circulatory systems of the brain. This channel connects the distal internal carotid, anterior, and posterior cerebral arteries via the anterior and posterior communicating arteries. The size of the circle of Willis is slightly larger than a quarter, and it resembles the shape of a hexagon. The circle of Willis is prone to congenital anomalies such as the development of a partial network in roughly 50% of patients, and many of the vessels are not symmetrical in size when compared to the contralateral side. In patients who do have a complete channel, it can serve as a collateral conduit in case one of the arteries on either the right or left side becomes blocked. The anterior and posterior communicating arteries serve as important collaterals if the extracranial arterial segments demonstrate significant stenosis.

Evaluation of the ACA with TCD

The anterior cerebral artery (ACA) begins when the distal ICA bifurcates within the cranium. These vessels are found bilaterally and are part of the anterior cerebrovascular system that supplies oxygenated blood to the brain and forms part of the circle of Willis. When assessing the ACA with transcranial Doppler (TCD), it is important to find the best window to insonate the vessel of interest. The transtemporal window may be used to evaluate the flow within the ACA, and from this level, normal flow should be away from the transducer because it is moving to the front of the patient's brain. The mean velocity of blood flow in the ACA is 50 ± 11 cm/s.

Blood Flow in a Normal MCA Using TCD

The bifurcation of the intracranial portion of the distal ICA gives way to two vessels: the MCA and the ACA. The MCA is the bigger of the two divisions that is part of the anterior cerebrovascular system. The MCA supplies blood to the lateral portions of the brain. Due to the location of the MCA, the best window during a TCD will be the transtemporal window. The transducer is placed on the side of the patient's head, and the first tracing encountered is usually the MCA. The direction of blood flow at this point should be toward the transducer. The velocity of a normal MCA will be 55 ± 12 cm/s.

Window Used to Insonate the PCA Using TCD

The posterior cerebral arteries (PCAs) are bilateral vessels that are formed from the bifurcation of the basilar artery to supply the occipital lobe and a portion of the temporal lobes of the brain with oxygenated blood. The PCAs help complete the circle of Willis and can be evaluated via the temporal window with TCD. To find the PCA, it may be helpful to find where the distal ICA splits into the middle and ACAs and angle the transducer posteriorly and inferiorly. Because the PCA curves, the waveform will first be directed toward the probe and then course away from the transducer in the second part of the vessel. The velocity of the PCA is normally 40 ± 10 cm/s.

Pseudoaneurysm

A pseudoaneurysm can result from any endovascular procedure, angiography, or the use of a dialysis access site. These are formed when blood seeps out of the artery and into the neighboring tissues. Patients may complain of a pulsatile, painful mass that appears red. The neck of this "false aneurysm" is the pathway that allows the blood to escape from the artery into the main capsule. Although some of these will resolve on their own, others will require procedures to create a clot. Some options for treatment include ultrasound-guided manual compression and injections. When injections are used, thrombin is instilled into the pocket to create a hematoma. Surgical repair is warranted when the artery is greatly damaged.

Copyright © Mometrix Media. You have been licensed one copy of this document for personal use only. Any other reproduction or redistribution is strictly prohibited. All rights reserved.
This content is provided for test preparation purposes only and does not imply an endorsement by Mometrix of any particular political, scientific, or religious point of view.

Amaurosis Fugax

The ophthalmic artery is the first branch of the ICA and is extremely important because it and all of its branches supplies the eye with the necessary blood flow. If a patient has ulcerated plaque within their ICA, one of the risks is a thromboembolic event that can create the effect of a shade that has dropped down over the eye or part of the eye and interferes with the patient's vision. This blindness that the patient experiences is temporary (often lasting 30 minutes or less), and the affected ophthalmic artery is on the same side as the diseased ICA in which the embolus traveled from and is characterized as a monocular episode.

Cerebrovascular Accident

A cerebrovascular accident (CVA) is the medical term for a stroke, which is a medical emergency. A stroke occurs because of an interruption of blood flow to the brain or if a blood vessel ruptures. Ischemic strokes are the most common type (approximately 85%), which happens when a blood clot forms in an artery that supplies the brain with blood (referred to as a thrombotic stroke). Another cause of an ischemic stroke is when a thrombus organizes in a different part of the body but breaks off and ends up in a smaller artery within the brain (known as an embolic stroke). The other 15% of strokes are hemorrhagic in nature, which may be from an aneurysm or other cause of bleeding in the brain. Although occurring less often, hemorrhagic strokes are often fatal.

Occluded Artery When a CVA Occurs

A CVA is an interruption of blood flow to the brain either due to an occlusion or a rupture of a blood vessel such as an aneurysm. The MCA is the cerebral artery that is occluded more than others to cause a stroke, otherwise known as a large-vessel stroke. The MCA stems from the ICA and takes a more lateral direction to supply the temporal, parietal, and frontal lobes of the brain with oxygenated blood. A CVA caused by the occlusion (or a possible bleed) of the MCA may result in numbness on the contralateral side of the body of the patient. Hemiplegia is also another symptom that the individual may experience.

Vasospasm and Typical Findings

A vasospasm causes the arteries in the body to contract, which greatly diminishes the amount of blood flow to the organs. Vasospasms can happen in all regions of the body, but when they occur in the brain, it is often the result of a ruptured brain aneurysm that created a subarachnoid hemorrhage. This hemorrhaging causes the arteries within the brain to contract; often, a couple of days later the complication of vasospasm sets in. TCD can be used to evaluate the velocity of the cerebral arteries and determine if vasospasm is present. A higher velocity within the cerebral arteries equals a greater chance of brain damage. Vasospasm usually maxes out around one to two weeks after the subarachnoid hemorrhage occurred and is noticeable in the cerebral arteries that are more prominent such as the MCA.

Temporal Arteritis

Vasculitis can be defined as the swelling of blood vessels. Temporal arteritis is one kind of vasculitis that occurs when the distal portion of the superficial temporal artery becomes inflamed. The external carotid arteries give rise to the temporal vessels, which are found near the temples of the patient and supply the scalp with oxygenated blood. The temporal artery divides into the frontal and parietal branches, which may also be affected. Although this is an extremely difficult diagnosis to make with ultrasound, the vessel will appear narrowed and edema may surround the lumen of the artery on gray-scale and color Doppler imaging. This condition is often diagnosed in women that are older than age 50; it is important to diagnose temporal arteritis quickly because the patient's vision may be lost if the arteries that supply blood to the eye are also affected.

Copyright © Mometrix Media. You have been licensed one copy of this document for personal use only. Any other reproduction or redistribution is strictly prohibited. All rights reserved.
This content is provided for test preparation purposes only and does not imply an endorsement by Mometrix of any particular political, scientific, or religious point of view.

Reasons for Another Carotid Duplex to Be Ordered

In most cases, it is believed to be unnecessary to perform another carotid duplex exam on the same patient unless that individual has experienced additional symptoms in which the physician wants to have the carotid duplex exam repeated in order to better treat the patient. Some of the things that a patient may report as worsening symptoms and affect the anterior circulation are problems speaking and amaurosis fugax. Symptoms that affect the posterior circulation include double vision and dysphagia with or without vertigo. If it has been established that a patient has experienced moderate (50%–69%) stenosis, they should undergo a follow-up study every year. For those that have severe (70%–99%) stenosis, it is recommended that a follow-up ultrasound should be performed every six months.

Effect of Calcifications on Carotid Duplex Exams

Calcifications are the result of calcium buildup within the wall of the artery. During ultrasound exams, plaque that is calcified appears as bright echoes that will often display posterior shadowing. This acoustic shadowing can be problematic because it can hinder the examination of the entire artery. If the vascular technologist attempts to estimate the percentage of stenosis in the presence of shadowing, errors will likely occur during the calculations. However, it may be beneficial for the sonographer to try to change the method used to access the vessels that are difficult to visualize well when there is a significant amount of shadowing present. For example, the vascular technologist may be able to access the vessel from a more posterior or anterior approach.

Ophthalmic Artery

The internal carotid artery (ICA) originates at the bifurcation of the CCA in the neck. The ICA has several branches to carry oxygenated blood to the brain and eyes. Typically, during a carotid duplex ultrasound, the divisions of the ICA are not seen because the divisions are not extracranial (recall that the branches of the ECA, however, can be seen in the neck). The first major intracranial division of the ICA is the ophthalmic artery, which supplies the eye with oxygenated blood. The ophthalmic artery is often seen at the curve of the ICA known as the carotid siphon, and it has several branches that supply various parts of the eye, the muscles that move the eyeball, as well as the eyelid. Notably, some of the arteries that stem from the ophthalmic artery connect with some of the ECA branches and may act as collateral channels if the ICA is diseased.

Spectral Waveform When Interrogating a Normal ICA

The ICA is one of two branches of the CCA found in the neck. The ICA is the blood vessel that transports the majority of the blood from the CCA to the brain. Because the function of the ICA is to supply the anterior and middle regions of the brain with oxygenated blood, it does so by its two terminal segments known as the anterior cerebral and middle cerebral arteries. The typical spectral waveform of a normal ICA will demonstrate a low-resistance, monophasic waveform when evaluated with spectral Doppler. Blood flow within the ICA should also be noted as continuous flow through diastole.

Discerning Between the ICA or ECA

When performing a carotid duplex exam, there are several elements that may help the vascular technologist discern between the ICA and ECA. It is important to understand the location of these vessels and to consider what organs or tissues they supply. For example, the ECA supplies oxygenated blood to the face, scalp, and neck and tends to be situated more medially than the ICA. The ICA provides blood flow to the brain and is found in a more lateral position of the neck. The ECA has several extracranial branches that can be seen during the exam in comparison to the ICA, which only has intracranial branches. Along with the branches, the ECA is typically smaller

Copyright © Mometrix Media. You have been licensed one copy of this document for personal use only. Any other reproduction or redistribution is strictly prohibited. All rights reserved.
This content is provided for test preparation purposes only and does not imply an endorsement by Mometrix of any particular political, scientific, or religious point of view.

compared to the ICA. However, the most dependable method is to use spectral Doppler. The ECA will demonstrate a rapid upstroke and downstroke during systole, less flow in diastole, and high-resistance blood flow in comparison to the ICA, which will demonstrate a waveform that is of low resistance.

Spectral Waveform When Performing a Carotid Duplex Study

The CCA supplies oxygenated blood to the head and neck regions. Most of the blood that travels through the CCA is directed into the ICA, which continuously feeds the brain with oxygenated blood. The continual supply of blood must occur amid the entire cardiac cycle, so a normal CCA should have a tracing that displays a moderately broad systolic peak as well as a moderate amount of diastolic flow. However, the blood that does not enter the ICA moves into the ECA, so the CCA has characteristics of both vessels that results in low- and high-resistance flow.

Blood Flow in the Posterolateral Portion of the Carotid Bulb

The carotid bulb is found in the distal portion of the CCA before the artery bifurcates into the ICA and the ECA. The carotid bulb is also referred to as the carotid sinus and is an area in which a noticeable dilation of the blood vessel may be visualized in the region of or just prior to the carotid bifurcation. When arteries are straight, the blood flow tends to display laminar flow. However, even without the presence of disease, the natural curve of the carotid bulb can cause a disturbance of flow in which separation occurs. The diameter of the carotid bulb as well as the divergence of the ICA and ECA origins can attribute to more pronounced flow separations.

Flow Characteristics of a Vertebral Artery That Is Unremarkable

The paired vertebral arteries ascend from the subclavian arteries on both sides of the neck to pass through the foramen magnum to eventually join to form the basilar artery. The basilar artery helps to supply the posterior region of the brain with oxygenated blood. The brain must have blood delivered to it continuously, so the flow patterns in the vertebral arteries should demonstrate low-resistance flow with continuous flow during diastole similar to that seen in the ICA because it also supplies the brain. The Doppler tracing should demonstrate flow that is moving toward the brain (antegrade).

Middle Cerebral Artery

The ICA enters the cranium on the right and left sides where it eventually bifurcates into the anterior cerebral arteries (ACAs) as well as the middle cerebral arteries (MCAs) at the terminal intracranial portion of the ICA. The MCA follows a more lateral projection in order to feed the cerebral cortex on the lateral sides of the brain. The MCA is often greater in diameter when compared to the ACA, and it is part of the anterior cerebrovascular circulatory system that supplies the brain with oxygenated blood. It is important for vascular technologists to realize that a large percentage of cerebrovascular accidents (CVAs) occur because the MCA has a high occlusion rate.

Depths and Velocities of Vessels

Terminal internal carotid artery (tICA), anterior cerebral artery (ACA), middle cerebral artery (MCA), posterior cerebral artery (PCA):

Artery	Direction of blood flow in comparison to the transducer	Depth	Normal velocity
tICA	Toward and/or away	60–70 mm	39 ± 9 cm/s
ACA	Away	60–75 mm	50 ± 11 cm/s

Copyright © Mometrix Media. You have been licensed one copy of this document for personal use only. Any other reproduction or redistribution is strictly prohibited. All rights reserved.
This content is provided for test preparation purposes only and does not imply an endorsement by Mometrix of any particular political, scientific, or religious point of view.

Artery	Direction of blood flow in comparison to the transducer	Depth	Normal velocity
MCA	First segment toward; second segment away	30–60 mm	55 ± 12 cm/s
PCA	First segment toward; second segment away	60–75 mm	40 ± 10 cm/s

Prevailing Vessel in Which Atherosclerosis Develops

In healthy patients, arteries demonstrate elasticity to move the blood throughout the circulatory system with the contractions of the heart. Arteriosclerosis takes place when the arterial walls no longer have the same elasticity. Atherosclerosis can be defined as plaque accumulation within the arteries due to damage to the arterial wall. This plaque can be comprised of cholesterol or fats and can restrict the flow of oxygen-rich blood to vital organs. Risk factors of arterial disease include smoking, hypertension, diabetes, high cholesterol, and high triglycerides. These plaques can also break off or erupt, initiating a DVT. Atherosclerosis can develop in any artery, but this condition typically occurs in the brachiocephalic vessel, carotid bifurcation, infrarenal aorta, and iliac and femoral arteries. Atherosclerosis is visualized in the distal femoral artery more often than in other arteries.

Appearance of the Waveform in the Right CCA

A carotid duplex ultrasound exam is a reliable, noninvasive exam used to determine the patency and direction of blood flow within various arteries. Spectral Doppler is an important component of a carotid duplex exam because each artery has a typical appearance (which will fluctuate a bit based on each patient that is examined) based on which organs and tissues are being supplied. For example, the CCA will demonstrate diastolic flow of moderate proportions and low-resistance flow as the majority of the blood continues into the ICA, which feeds the brain. When a distal occlusion is present and the right ICA is occluded, there will be less diastolic flow, which is created when there is more resistance. If the right ICA is completely occluded, then it would not be surprising to see an absence of flow within the right CCA.

Scenarios for Turbulent Blood Flow

The type of blood flow that makes up the majority of flow dynamics within the blood vessels of the human body is known as laminar flow. During laminar flow, red blood cells within the center of the vessel are moving faster than those in the outer walls in a more layered appearance. Turbulence is considered to be flow that is not orderly or layered such as that found in laminar flow. Turbulent flow is often noted distal to a segment of vessel that is stenotic, but this type of blood flow is also evident in blood vessels that are not diseased and may even be considered normal in some arteries. Turbulent flow may be noticed in patients that have vessels that are tortuous or when the artery is kinked. Turbulence may also be witnessed when the artery becomes expanded, such as in the region of the carotid bulb.

Scenario

During a carotid duplex study, if color flow demonstrates blood flow in the carotid bulb but not the ICA, discuss what the vascular technologist may assume and how to continue the exam.

During a carotid duplex study, if the vascular technologist can obtain color flow in the carotid bulb, but not in the ICA, then it should be assumed that the ICA is totally occluded. However, it is important to continue the exam by using continuous-wave and/or pulsed-wave Doppler in addition to gray-scale, color, and power Doppler. The vascular technologist should make several attempts to

Copyright © Mometrix Media. You have been licensed one copy of this document for personal use only. Any other reproduction or redistribution is strictly prohibited. All rights reserved.
This content is provided for test preparation purposes only and does not imply an endorsement by Mometrix of any particular political, scientific, or religious point of view.

determine flow because the patient is managed differently depending on whether the diagnosis is total or occlusion or a critical stenosis. Patients with a severe stenosis may be candidates for a carotid endarterectomy, but this is not the case when the ICA is totally occluded. Ultrasound is often the first study performed if carotid artery disease is suspected, but it may be followed up with a magnetic resonance angiogram or a carotid angiogram, which is a more invasive test.

Typical Location of Atherosclerosis

Atherosclerosis is a disease that progresses over time and is one of the leading causes of strokes and heart attacks. With this condition, plaque tends to create a narrowing of the blood vessels, which can limit the amount of blood flow to vital organs. Plaque is the result of a buildup of fat and cholesterol in an artery that can create a thickening of the intima of the arterial wall. Sometimes, this thickening extends into the middle layer in addition to the inner layer. This accumulation of plaque can create a narrowing of the artery known as stenosis. During a carotid duplex exam, the vascular technologist will often locate atherosclerosis at the bifurcation of the carotid artery, especially where the ICA branches from the CCA.

Inaccurate Measurements from a Pulsed-Wave Doppler

Pulsed-wave Doppler is a useful method to measure blood flow velocities within various blood vessels. The ultrasound user has the option to select where the gate should be placed within a vessel in order to take a velocity measurement and know the exact location of this reading. However, sometimes, the velocity within the blood vessel is too high and the sonographer is unable to obtain an accurate peak velocity measurement. The sonographer would want to switch to continuous-wave Doppler because velocities that are extremely high tend to be more accurate because there isn't a maximum velocity while using this method. While using pulsed-wave Doppler, if the user cannot eliminate aliasing after trying to change the scale, the depth of the target, and switching to a lower frequency probe, then he or she can switch to continuous-wave Doppler.

Carotid Dissection

A carotid dissection occurs when the tunica intima (inner) layer of the arterial wall is torn, which enables blood to get between the layers of the arterial wall. Much like an aortic dissection, a false lumen develops and can expand in both directions, which may cause an obstruction. The sonographic visualization of an intimal flap in the carotid artery can help diagnose a carotid dissection. It is important to note that the blood within the false lumen may clot or even embolize, which can lead to a stroke. Color and spectral Doppler may demonstrate blood flowing in opposite directions in the false and true lumens. Spectral Doppler signals may also show different velocities on either side of the intimal flap. Carotid dissections are typically the result of trauma such as a motorcycle or car accident, especially in the younger population. Spontaneous dissections have been reported, although they are not as common. Individuals with connective tissue disorders such as Marfan syndrome or Ehlers-Danlos syndrome are at a slightly higher risk of a dissection.

Types and Appearances of Atherosclerotic Plaque

During a carotid duplex exam, vascular technologists will encounter various types and appearances of atherosclerotic plaque within the carotid arteries. Clinicians can use ultrasound as a predictive tool to help determine individuals that have the greatest risk of a stroke by evaluating who has plaque that appears suspicious for hemorrhage or ulceration. If the lesion contains plaque that consists of fibrous tissue, calcium, cellular particles, and collagen, it is referred to as a complicated lesion, which often takes on a heterogenous appearance. An ulcerative plaque is especially concerning because particles may break off and become lodged in a distal artery causing a transient ischemic attack, or stroke. This is considered an unstable plaque because the surface of the lesion begins to break down to allow the contents within to possibly escape. An intraplaque hemorrhage is

Copyright © Mometrix Media. You have been licensed one copy of this document for personal use only. Any other reproduction or redistribution is strictly prohibited. All rights reserved.
This content is provided for test preparation purposes only and does not imply an endorsement by Mometrix of any particular political, scientific, or religious point of view.

identified when a low-level echogenic component is seen within a plaque. This condition also puts the patient at a greater risk of embolism if there is a rupture.

Carotid Endarterectomy

A carotid endarterectomy is a procedure in which the surgeon exposes the lumen of the carotid artery in order to visualize and remove plaque that has accumulated within the vessel. This procedure is performed to reduce the risk of an ischemic stroke. Often, patients present to the ultrasound lab not because they are symptomatic, but rather their physician detected a carotid bruit, which suggests carotid stenosis. Other patients describe transient ischemic attack symptoms such as a temporary loss of vision, speech, weakness, or numbness that occurs unilaterally. Patients that undergo this type of surgery must be watched closely for complications such as breathing issues if the trachea is compressed by a hematoma that has developed, bleeding of the incision, or neointimal hyperplasia. Neointimal hyperplasia is often responsible for restenosis between 6 and 24 months postoperative because there is rapid growth of the smooth muscle cells as the tissue is attempting to heal. Notably, this procedure is not performed when a complete occlusion of the ICA has been proven.

Abnormal Sound in the Neck

When a healthcare provider uses the stethoscope to listen to a patient's neck and hears an abnormal sound, it is referred to as a bruit. Laminar flow is the typical blood flow pattern, but a bruit that occurs when this pattern is no longer present is often the result of turbulent blood flow such as in the case of a carotid stenosis. However, providers must not rely on the presence or absence of an audible bruit to diagnose disease. If a bruit is heard and it continues in diastole, the provider will be especially concerned because this is indicative of a significant stenosis of 70%–80% lumen diameter reduction. If a bruit was previously heard in a patient but is no longer present, this likely means that the diameter reduction is now more than 90% and the disease classification is now considered to be preocclusive.

Obtaining Reliable Measurement of the PSV

Often during a carotid duplex exam, a vascular technologist will notice an incidental cardiac arrhythmia on a patient. This does not typically pose a problem during the exam, and it is possible to obtain a reliable measurement of the PSV once the sinus rhythm becomes normal again. Ultrasound protocols may vary from one lab to another in patients that have a severe cardiac arrhythmia because attaining PSV measurements can often be difficult. It may be advantageous to obtain a ratio of the highest measured PSV of the ICA and compare it to the distal CCA PSV. Interpreting physicians may request that the vascular technologist averages 3 or 4 cycles (although some will require up to 10 cycles) as the preferred protocol in cases of severe arrhythmias.

Abnormality Visualized in the Circle of Willis

The circle of Willis is an arterial ring that is comprised of segments of the anterior and posterior intracranial blood vessels. This structure is about the same diameter of a 50-cent piece and sits at the base of the brain. The blood vessels that are part of the circle of Willis are the distal internal carotid, anterior cerebral, posterior cerebral, and communicating arteries. Although the name suggests that this connection is complete, less than 50% of the population has a circle of Willis that is fully developed. One of the most common abnormalities of this structure is the lack of at least one of the two communicating arteries. Having a circle of Willis that is fully developed is advantageous if the patient develops a significant stenosis or blockage and it can serve as a collateral channel.

Copyright © Mometrix Media. You have been licensed one copy of this document for personal use only. Any other reproduction or redistribution is strictly prohibited. All rights reserved.
This content is provided for test preparation purposes only and does not imply an endorsement by Mometrix of any particular political, scientific, or religious point of view.

Carotid Body Tumor

A carotid body tumor is a rare finding that may be visualized when a vascular technologist is performing a carotid duplex exam on a patient or if the patient presents with a palpable neck mass. If a mass is identified that demonstrates an extreme amount of vascularity and is situated between the ECA and the ICA, then the vascular technologist should suspect a carotid body tumor. These masses are typically supplied with blood from the ECA and tend to grow slowly, but over time they can develop into a prominent mass. The patient may notice a pulsatile mass in the upper region of the neck, difficulty swallowing, neck and shoulder pain, as well as modifications in vision and blood pressure. Typically, symptoms do not manifest until the tumor becomes sizable. Although rarely cancerous, treatment of carotid body tumors includes radiation therapy, surgical excision, and embolization.

Masses Visualized During a Carotid Duplex Study

It is not uncommon for a vascular technologist to visualize masses in the neck while performing a carotid duplex study. For example, the patient may have enlarged lymph nodes that are apparent, especially if the patient has been sick recently. Medial to the carotid arteries is the thyroid gland, which is a butterfly-shaped gland located in the middle of the neck. It is not uncommon to find solid and cystic masses. Cysts contain fluid and are typically benign. Multinodular goiters are another common finding of the thyroid gland, which creates an enlarged thyroid. Nodules can be inflammatory if the patient has Hashimoto's disease, and other solid nodules may be present as well. Large masses can quickly be measured and documented as an incidental finding.

Vertebral Arteries

The right and left subclavian arteries serve as the origin of the right and left vertebral arteries. The vertebral arteries travel superiorly in the neck as the first division of the subclavian arteries in a more posterior position than the ICA. In fact, starting with the foramen of the sixth cervical (C6) vertebra, the vertebral arteries continue to pass through the foramina of the more superior cervical vertebrae to travel upward toward the base of the skull to enter the foramen magnum, which is found in the posterior portion of the skull. The foramen magnum is a large opening in the occipital bone that allows the brain stem and spinal cord to unite. These arteries join to form the basilar artery, which supplies oxygenated blood to the posterior structures of the brain. The vertebral arteries are not typically the same size because the left vertebral artery is often slightly larger than the right.

Window Used During TCD to Visualize the Vertebral Arteries

Recall that the vertebral arteries are situated in a more posterior location as they move superiorly from the clavicles toward the brain, passing through the cervical transverse foramen. To access the posterior region, it is helpful to use the suboccipital window. This can be obtained by having the patient roll onto his or her side facing away from the sonographer and asking the patient to tuck their chin toward the chest. The transducer can be placed on the middle of the posterior neck just below the skull. The sonographer can then angle the beam up through the foramen magnum to better visualize the vertebral arteries. The vertebral arteries take on the appearance of a V shape before they unite to become the basilar artery. Flow in the vertebral arteries should move in a direction away from the transducer. The basilar artery can also be examined via the suboccipital window.

Pathway of Blood After It Reaches the Right and Left Innominate Veins

The right and left innominate veins, also known as the brachiocephalic veins, are formed by the confluence of the internal jugular vein in the neck and the subclavian vein. The right innominate

Copyright © Mometrix Media. You have been licensed one copy of this document for personal use only. Any other reproduction or redistribution is strictly prohibited. All rights reserved.
This content is provided for test preparation purposes only and does not imply an endorsement by Mometrix of any particular political, scientific, or religious point of view.

vein receives blood from the right side of their body above the level of the heart to include the brain, neck, and right arm via the subclavian vein, whereas the left innominate vein receives blood from the left side of the body above the level of the heart to include the brain, neck, and left arm via the subclavian vein. The left innominate vein is longer than the right because it needs to reach the right atrium of the heart. The right and left innominate veins merge to form the superior vena cava (SVC). The SVC dumps deoxygenated blood into the right atrium of the heart.

Subclavian Arteries

There are two subclavian arteries (one on each side of the body), and it is important to note that the origins of the right and left subclavian arteries are very different. The right subclavian artery is the result of the bifurcation of the innominate (brachiocephalic) artery, which is the first division of the aortic arch that originates from the right side. The innominate artery bifurcates and branches into the right CCA as well as the right subclavian artery. The left subclavian artery stems from the arch of the aorta and is the third vessel to stem from the arch. The subclavian arteries give off several branches with the vertebral artery being one of the arteries that vascular technologists will interrogate during carotid duplex exams. The subclavian arteries are found just above the clavicles and becomes the axillary artery upon reaching the ribs.

Left CCA and the Left Subclavian Artery

The aortic arch contains three significant branches. The left CCA supplies oxygenated blood to the left side of the brain, face, and neck and is the second branch of the aortic arch. Vascular technologists can follow the left CCA from the bottom of the neck in a cephalad direction to the carotid bifurcation. The right CCA, on the other hand, does not branch directly from the aortic arch, but rather from the innominate artery, which is the first vessel to branch from the arch. The left subclavian artery is the third branch of the arch. This vessel carries oxygenated blood to the left upper extremity and branches several times to also supply blood to the chest. From the aortic arch, it passes above the clavicle to the lateral portion of the first rib to become the axillary artery.

Internal Thoracic Artery May Require Mapping

The subclavian artery has several branches, one of which is the internal thoracic artery. This artery is also referred to as the internal mammary artery, and it arises near the origin of the subclavian artery to descend along both sides of the sternum to supply oxygenated blood to the breasts and anterior wall of the thoracic cavity. This artery is often used by plastic surgeons in patients that have had a mastectomy as a microvascular anastomosis for transverse rectus abdominis myocutaneous flaps when patients have chosen to undergo breast reconstruction. Ultrasound can be used to determine patency and the size of the artery. The diameter of this artery should be 2 mm and should demonstrate low-resistance flow. Cardiothoracic surgeons may also use the internal thoracic artery when a coronary artery bypass surgery is necessary. The internal thoracic artery is often chosen because this type of graft has less risk of becoming occluded than grafts created by veins. The left internal thoracic artery is often used because of the close proximity to the heart.

Paget-Schroetter Syndrome

Thoracic outlet syndrome (TOS) may occur due to compression (or clotting) of veins, arteries, or nerves in the small area between the clavicle and first rib, which is known as the thoracic outlet. If this space tends to be more narrow than usual, compression of these structures and venous stasis can occur. Paget-Schroetter syndrome is part of the venous component of TOS and is typically created when the subclavian or axillary vein becomes clotted due to activities that involve the same or exaggerated motions of the upper extremities. Often, sports-related activities create repetitive movements that can stress these blood vessels and create a clot such as swimming, throwing a football or baseball, or lifting weights. Other non-sports-related injuries occur when people

Copyright © Mometrix Media. You have been licensed one copy of this document for personal use only. Any other reproduction or redistribution is strictly prohibited. All rights reserved.
This content is provided for test preparation purposes only and does not imply an endorsement by Mometrix of any particular political, scientific, or religious point of view.

constantly lift or hold heavy items overhead or work on computers without giving their body the proper amount of time to rest. Paget-Schroetter syndrome is also referred to as stress or effort thrombosis; symptoms include pain in the shoulder or arm with or without numbness or tingling. People may also complain of weakness of the affected hand when trying to grab objects.

Flow Patterns When Examining the Subclavian Veins

The subclavian veins are found on each side of the body. The subclavian veins originate near the first rib once the axillary and cephalic veins merge. As the name implies, the subclavian vein travels underneath the clavicle and is anterior to the subclavian artery. The subclavian vein tends to demonstrate pulsatile venous flow due to a location that is in close proximity to the heart. Along with cardiac pulsations, veins that are situated closer to the heart also demonstrate respiratory patterns. The internal jugular, brachiocephalic, and subclavian veins all have similar waveforms. As the vessels travel further away from the heart such as those found in the lower extremities, the vessels are compressible (as long as there is not a blood clot) and have spontaneous, phasic flow. When the distal extremity is squeezed, augmentation will be exhibited.

No Demonstration of Pulsatile Flow

Vascular technologists should expect to see pulsatile flow when evaluating the subclavian vein with spectral Doppler. This pulsatility occurs because the subclavian vein is positioned close to the heart. If the subclavian vein does not demonstrate phasic, pulsatile flow, then it is assumed that there is an obstruction proximal to the subclavian vein on the side being evaluated. Often, the flow in this case will become continuous in addition to the loss of pulsatility. Due to the bony anatomy around the subclavian and brachiocephalic veins, it can be difficult to perform compression when ruling out a DVT, so it is important to use color and spectral Doppler for evaluation, which is why it is important to understand the normal waveforms of veins that are close to the heart. Always evaluate for the presence of echogenic material within the lumen of the blood vessel as well as collaterals that may have developed.

Signs to Aid in the Diagnosis of TOS

Thoracic outlet syndrome (TOS) may occur due to factors related to arterial or venous complications. Although roughly 30% of people with TOS do not experience any symptoms, others present with pain in the shoulder or upper arm further accompanied by numbness and/or tingling. Other individuals may notice a decrease in the force of their grip. Patients may notice that this pain or numbness intensifies when working out, especially when their arm is in certain raised positions. Vascular technologists should prove that flow is at least reduced (because it is not always absent) when scanning the patient in different positions. Notably, the patient may be suffering from disorders related to the cervical spine or carpal tunnel because they may provoke similar symptoms.

Subclavian Steal Syndrome

The vertebral arteries are a conduit for blood flow to the brain. In cases of a subclavian steal, the blood travels to the arm instead of the brain on the affected side. This is due to a stenosis or even total occlusion in a location that is proximal to the vertebral artery (such as in the innominate or subclavian artery). The origin of the left subclavian artery is the aortic arch, so this is a condition that is seen more often on the left side. If the blood pressure is measured on both arms, the systolic component of the affected side is at least 15–20 mmHg less than the other side. Ultrasound will demonstrate a reversal of flow in the ipsilateral vertebral artery if there is complete occlusion of the subclavian artery. If the proximal vessels are not completely occluded, then the waveforms can vary depending on the amount of stenosis and can vary from early systolic deceleration to bidirectional flow as the stenosis becomes more advanced. The diagram demonstrates the blood

Copyright © Mometrix Media. You have been licensed one copy of this document for personal use only. Any other reproduction or redistribution is strictly prohibited. All rights reserved.
This content is provided for test preparation purposes only and does not imply an endorsement by Mometrix of any particular political, scientific, or religious point of view.

from the right vertebral artery moving into the left vertebral artery to help supply the left arm because the proximal left subclavian artery is occluded.

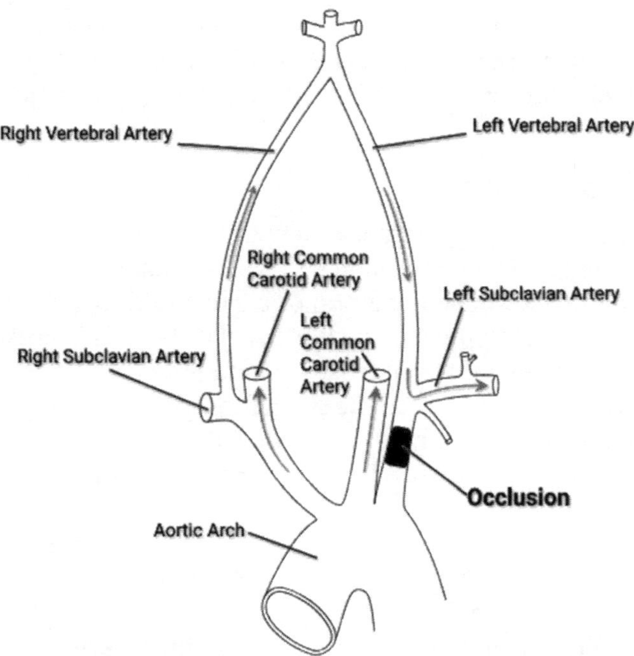

Myointimal Hyperplasia

Myointimal hyperplasia is concerning for an individual that has had a lower extremity bypass surgery performed because when stenosis develops in the first two years after the creation of a bypass graft it usually does so because of this condition. The area of the valve site is the typical location for the formation of stenosis. Myointimal hyperplasia can have a negative effect after bypass surgery because it can cause a blockage. Myointimal hyperplasia is the result of trauma to the endothelial cells after a grafting has taken place in which cells from the middle layer of the wall move to the inner layer and multiply and create a buildup when mixed with extracellular matrix, lymphocytes, and macrophages. This proliferation of cells can become problematic and lead to the constriction of the lumen of the blood vessel and hamper blood flow.

Indications for a Postoperative Hemodialysis Access

Due to the high failure rate postoperatively within the first year for postoperative hemodialysis access, ultrasound imaging may be necessary to aid clinicians to determine if the access site is functioning even when the clinical exam appears normal. Common indications for an ultrasound evaluation of the hemodialysis access site is if a blood flow rate of 400 mL/min cannot be achieved or if bleeding occurs longer than expected post dialysis even when pressure is applied. Another indication for imaging is if the AVF does not mature even after at least six weeks. An ultrasound will be ordered postoperatively if the patient has pain or swelling or has a cold hand or fingers after having dialysis or after the surgery has taken place. If a thrill cannot be felt over a fistula or if it appears to be smaller than expected, then an ultrasound evaluation should be performed.

Stenosis Is Suspected in an Upper Extremity AVF

If stenosis of an upper extremity AVF is suspected, the vascular technologist has several steps to complete because the fistula along with the anastomosis, draining vein, arterial inflow, as well as evaluate for any fluid collections should be done. The diameter of the fistula should be the first

Copyright © Mometrix Media. You have been licensed one copy of this document for personal use only. Any other reproduction or redistribution is strictly prohibited. All rights reserved.
This content is provided for test preparation purposes only and does not imply an endorsement by Mometrix of any particular political, scientific, or religious point of view.

thing that is documented, and this can be evaluated with gray-scale ultrasound. The PSV ratio of the anastomosis/artery 2 cm upstream should be calculated as well. The draining vein should be assessed with gray-scale, color, and spectral Doppler. Stenosis or even thrombosis is suspected of the cranial system if there is little to no flow in the draining vein. Once again, the PSV ratio is calculated, but this time it is the comparison of the narrowed draining vein to the vein 2 cm upstream. The subclavian and internal jugular veins should be examined with spectral Doppler to check for stenosis as well. Although stenosis of the inflow artery is fairly unusual, the feeding artery should also be evaluated.

AVF That Has Failed to Mature

When scanning a patient postoperatively because their AVF has not matured even after four to eight weeks post surgery, the goal is to determine if there is an anatomic issue that can be repaired. The anastomosis is scanned to determine if it is stenotic. The draining vein should be evaluated with gray-scale, color, and spectral Doppler as well to see if a stenosis is present. The diameter of the AVF should be measured and should be at least 4 mm in order for it to be functional. Volume blood flow measurements are taken as well in the straightest segment possible that does not show turbulence and is in the middle of the draining vein. Calculations of 500–600 mL/min tend to have a high affinity for a positive outcome for this AVF to use for hemodialysis.

Arteriovenous Fistula

The circulatory system is a closed network of blood vessels that carries oxygenated blood to the cells of the body and returns blood that has been depleted of oxygen back to the heart. The blood travels through the body once it is pumped from the heart to the arteries, arterioles, capillaries, venules, and then to the veins. If blood passes directly from the arteries to the veins, it is known as an arteriovenous fistula (AVF). When the atypical assembly of these vessels occurs, it is important to diagnose this condition as quickly as possible because the regions that are fed by the capillaries receives a reduced blood supply preventing them from obtaining the proper amounts of nutrients and oxygen. Individuals that are undergoing dialysis may need to have a procedure in which an AVF is generated so that it can be used as an access site. AVFs may materialize on their own or as the result of trauma.

Access Method for Dialysis

For individuals that will undergo dialysis, the access method that is preferred would be an arteriovenous fistula (AVF) of the nondominant forearm. If the forearm can be used, the connection that is favored is the brachial artery to cephalic vein route. The forearm is favored over the upper arm, but if the nondominant forearm cannot be used, then the dominant forearm may be the site of access. Sonographic evaluation of the AVF includes measuring the diameter of the fistula as well as the draining vein (this should be 4 mm or more) to help determine if narrowing of these structures has occurred. A PSV ratio of 2:1 results in at least a 50% stenosis of the AVF when the draining vein is compared to a point 2 cm upstream.

Provide Guidance for Thrombin Injections of Pseudoaneurysms

Ultrasound is not only a great modality to diagnose a pseudoaneurysm, but it is also a great tool to help monitor this pulsatile mass to determine if it will clot on its own. Sometimes surgical repair is necessary for pseudoaneurysms, but most of the time compression or percutaneous thrombin injections are useful, with thrombin injection being the most common procedure that is done. Gray-scale and color Doppler ultrasound are used during the injection process until it appears as if the pseudoaneurysm is clotted. Once there is an absence of flow when monitoring with color Doppler, it is assumed that thrombosis has taken place. The vascular technologist should also document images of the proximal and distal arteries of this pulsatile mass.

Copyright © Mometrix Media. You have been licensed one copy of this document for personal use only. Any other reproduction or redistribution is strictly prohibited. All rights reserved.
This content is provided for test preparation purposes only and does not imply an endorsement by Mometrix of any particular political, scientific, or religious point of view.

Evaluating the Liver If the Patient Has a TIPS

A transjugular intrahepatic portosystemic shunt is placed between the hepatic and portal veins to alleviate the pressure in the portal system that may be causing ascites or variceal bleeding. In patients that have severe portal hypertension, the flow of blood within the portal venous system tends to be in a hepatofugal direction (flowing away from the liver) instead of hepatopetal (flowing toward the liver). After the stent is placed, a baseline ultrasound should be performed to check the shunt with B-mode and color Doppler. When color Doppler is applied, the entire stent should demonstrate complete color filling. If the ultrasound operator does not see color flow, then one can assume that there is a blockage. If spectral waveforms demonstrate velocities that are extremely high or low when compared to the baseline exam, one may assume that there is a stenosis. Other indicators that the stent is no longer working correctly are a shift in directional flow within the portal vein, ascites that has increased, or the presence of collateral channels visualized with ultrasound.

Complications Incurred During TIPS Insertion

Following TIPS insertion, complications may occur even though there have been high overall success rates because this is a very technical procedure to complete. It is important for the patient to have labs and a complete abdominal ultrasound workup prior to TIPS insertion to establish a baseline and to prevent complications. One of the most serious postprocedure complications is acute liver failure. Fortunately, this does not occur very often, but when it does happen, it is associated with a poor outcome for the patient unless a liver transplant is performed. Another rare complication is hemorrhaging during a TIPS procedure. Symptoms that the patient may have are abdominal pain and distension, vomiting blood, or abnormal blood pressure. Various injuries of arteries have also been reported, which may result in the occlusion of the artery or formation of a pseudoaneurysm.

Copyright © Mometrix Media. You have been licensed one copy of this document for personal use only. Any other reproduction or redistribution is strictly prohibited. All rights reserved.
This content is provided for test preparation purposes only and does not imply an endorsement by Mometrix of any particular political, scientific, or religious point of view.

How to Overcome Test Anxiety

Just the thought of taking a test is enough to make most people a little nervous. A test is an important event that can have a long-term impact on your future, so it's important to take it seriously and it's natural to feel anxious about performing well. But just because anxiety is normal, that doesn't mean that it's helpful in test taking, or that you should simply accept it as part of your life. Anxiety can have a variety of effects. These effects can be mild, like making you feel slightly nervous, or severe, like blocking your ability to focus or remember even a simple detail.

If you experience test anxiety—whether severe or mild—it's important to know how to beat it. To discover this, first you need to understand what causes test anxiety.

Causes of Test Anxiety

While we often think of anxiety as an uncontrollable emotional state, it can actually be caused by simple, practical things. One of the most common causes of test anxiety is that a person does not feel adequately prepared for their test. This feeling can be the result of many different issues such as poor study habits or lack of organization, but the most common culprit is time management. Starting to study too late, failing to organize your study time to cover all of the material, or being distracted while you study will mean that you're not well prepared for the test. This may lead to cramming the night before, which will cause you to be physically and mentally exhausted for the test. Poor time management also contributes to feelings of stress, fear, and hopelessness as you realize you are not well prepared but don't know what to do about it.

Other times, test anxiety is not related to your preparation for the test but comes from unresolved fear. This may be a past failure on a test, or poor performance on tests in general. It may come from comparing yourself to others who seem to be performing better or from the stress of living up to expectations. Anxiety may be driven by fears of the future—how failure on this test would affect your educational and career goals. These fears are often completely irrational, but they can still negatively impact your test performance.

Review Video: 3 Reasons You Have Test Anxiety
Visit mometrix.com/academy and enter code: 428468

Copyright © Mometrix Media. You have been licensed one copy of this document for personal use only. Any other reproduction or redistribution is strictly prohibited. All rights reserved.
This content is provided for test preparation purposes only and does not imply an endorsement by Mometrix of any particular political, scientific, or religious point of view.

Elements of Test Anxiety

As mentioned earlier, test anxiety is considered to be an emotional state, but it has physical and mental components as well. Sometimes you may not even realize that you are suffering from test anxiety until you notice the physical symptoms. These can include trembling hands, rapid heartbeat, sweating, nausea, and tense muscles. Extreme anxiety may lead to fainting or vomiting. Obviously, any of these symptoms can have a negative impact on testing. It is important to recognize them as soon as they begin to occur so that you can address the problem before it damages your performance.

Review Video: 3 Ways to Tell You Have Test Anxiety
Visit mometrix.com/academy and enter code: 927847

The mental components of test anxiety include trouble focusing and inability to remember learned information. During a test, your mind is on high alert, which can help you recall information and stay focused for an extended period of time. However, anxiety interferes with your mind's natural processes, causing you to blank out, even on the questions you know well. The strain of testing during anxiety makes it difficult to stay focused, especially on a test that may take several hours. Extreme anxiety can take a huge mental toll, making it difficult not only to recall test information but even to understand the test questions or pull your thoughts together.

Review Video: How Test Anxiety Affects Memory
Visit mometrix.com/academy and enter code: 609003

Effects of Test Anxiety

Test anxiety is like a disease—if left untreated, it will get progressively worse. Anxiety leads to poor performance, and this reinforces the feelings of fear and failure, which in turn lead to poor performances on subsequent tests. It can grow from a mild nervousness to a crippling condition. If allowed to progress, test anxiety can have a big impact on your schooling, and consequently on your future.

Test anxiety can spread to other parts of your life. Anxiety on tests can become anxiety in any stressful situation, and blanking on a test can turn into panicking in a job situation. But fortunately, you don't have to let anxiety rule your testing and determine your grades. There are a number of relatively simple steps you can take to move past anxiety and function normally on a test and in the rest of life.

Review Video: How Test Anxiety Impacts Your Grades
Visit mometrix.com/academy and enter code: 939819

Copyright © Mometrix Media. You have been licensed one copy of this document for personal use only. Any other reproduction or redistribution is strictly prohibited. All rights reserved.
This content is provided for test preparation purposes only and does not imply an endorsement by Mometrix of any particular political, scientific, or religious point of view.

Physical Steps for Beating Test Anxiety

While test anxiety is a serious problem, the good news is that it can be overcome. It doesn't have to control your ability to think and remember information. While it may take time, you can begin taking steps today to beat anxiety.

Just as your first hint that you may be struggling with anxiety comes from the physical symptoms, the first step to treating it is also physical. Rest is crucial for having a clear, strong mind. If you are tired, it is much easier to give in to anxiety. But if you establish good sleep habits, your body and mind will be ready to perform optimally, without the strain of exhaustion. Additionally, sleeping well helps you to retain information better, so you're more likely to recall the answers when you see the test questions.

Getting good sleep means more than going to bed on time. It's important to allow your brain time to relax. Take study breaks from time to time so it doesn't get overworked, and don't study right before bed. Take time to rest your mind before trying to rest your body, or you may find it difficult to fall asleep.

Review Video: The Importance of Sleep for Your Brain
Visit mometrix.com/academy and enter code: 319338

Along with sleep, other aspects of physical health are important in preparing for a test. Good nutrition is vital for good brain function. Sugary foods and drinks may give a burst of energy but this burst is followed by a crash, both physically and emotionally. Instead, fuel your body with protein and vitamin-rich foods.

Also, drink plenty of water. Dehydration can lead to headaches and exhaustion, especially if your brain is already under stress from the rigors of the test. Particularly if your test is a long one, drink water during the breaks. And if possible, take an energy-boosting snack to eat between sections.

Review Video: How Diet Can Affect your Mood
Visit mometrix.com/academy and enter code: 624317

Along with sleep and diet, a third important part of physical health is exercise. Maintaining a steady workout schedule is helpful, but even taking 5-minute study breaks to walk can help get your blood pumping faster and clear your head. Exercise also releases endorphins, which contribute to a positive feeling and can help combat test anxiety.

When you nurture your physical health, you are also contributing to your mental health. If your body is healthy, your mind is much more likely to be healthy as well. So take time to rest, nourish your body with healthy food and water, and get moving as much as possible. Taking these physical steps will make you stronger and more able to take the mental steps necessary to overcome test anxiety.

Copyright © Mometrix Media. You have been licensed one copy of this document for personal use only. Any other reproduction or redistribution is strictly prohibited. All rights reserved.
This content is provided for test preparation purposes only and does not imply an endorsement by Mometrix of any particular political, scientific, or religious point of view.

Mental Steps for Beating Test Anxiety

Working on the mental side of test anxiety can be more challenging, but as with the physical side, there are clear steps you can take to overcome it. As mentioned earlier, test anxiety often stems from lack of preparation, so the obvious solution is to prepare for the test. Effective studying may be the most important weapon you have for beating test anxiety, but you can and should employ several other mental tools to combat fear.

First, boost your confidence by reminding yourself of past success—tests or projects that you aced. If you're putting as much effort into preparing for this test as you did for those, there's no reason you should expect to fail here. Work hard to prepare; then trust your preparation.

Second, surround yourself with encouraging people. It can be helpful to find a study group, but be sure that the people you're around will encourage a positive attitude. If you spend time with others who are anxious or cynical, this will only contribute to your own anxiety. Look for others who are motivated to study hard from a desire to succeed, not from a fear of failure.

Third, reward yourself. A test is physically and mentally tiring, even without anxiety, and it can be helpful to have something to look forward to. Plan an activity following the test, regardless of the outcome, such as going to a movie or getting ice cream.

When you are taking the test, if you find yourself beginning to feel anxious, remind yourself that you know the material. Visualize successfully completing the test. Then take a few deep, relaxing breaths and return to it. Work through the questions carefully but with confidence, knowing that you are capable of succeeding.

Developing a healthy mental approach to test taking will also aid in other areas of life. Test anxiety affects more than just the actual test—it can be damaging to your mental health and even contribute to depression. It's important to beat test anxiety before it becomes a problem for more than testing.

Review Video: Test Anxiety and Depression
Visit mometrix.com/academy and enter code: 904704

Copyright © Mometrix Media. You have been licensed one copy of this document for personal use only. Any other reproduction or redistribution is strictly prohibited. All rights reserved.
This content is provided for test preparation purposes only and does not imply an endorsement by Mometrix of any particular political, scientific, or religious point of view.

Study Strategy

Being prepared for the test is necessary to combat anxiety, but what does being prepared look like? You may study for hours on end and still not feel prepared. What you need is a strategy for test prep. The next few pages outline our recommended steps to help you plan out and conquer the challenge of preparation.

Step 1: Scope Out the Test

Learn everything you can about the format (multiple choice, essay, etc.) and what will be on the test. Gather any study materials, course outlines, or sample exams that may be available. Not only will this help you to prepare, but knowing what to expect can help to alleviate test anxiety.

Step 2: Map Out the Material

Look through the textbook or study guide and make note of how many chapters or sections it has. Then divide these over the time you have. For example, if a book has 15 chapters and you have five days to study, you need to cover three chapters each day. Even better, if you have the time, leave an extra day at the end for overall review after you have gone through the material in depth.

If time is limited, you may need to prioritize the material. Look through it and make note of which sections you think you already have a good grasp on, and which need review. While you are studying, skim quickly through the familiar sections and take more time on the challenging parts. Write out your plan so you don't get lost as you go. Having a written plan also helps you feel more in control of the study, so anxiety is less likely to arise from feeling overwhelmed at the amount to cover.

Step 3: Gather Your Tools

Decide what study method works best for you. Do you prefer to highlight in the book as you study and then go back over the highlighted portions? Or do you type out notes of the important information? Or is it helpful to make flashcards that you can carry with you? Assemble the pens, index cards, highlighters, post-it notes, and any other materials you may need so you won't be distracted by getting up to find things while you study.

If you're having a hard time retaining the information or organizing your notes, experiment with different methods. For example, try color-coding by subject with colored pens, highlighters, or post-it notes. If you learn better by hearing, try recording yourself reading your notes so you can listen while in the car, working out, or simply sitting at your desk. Ask a friend to quiz you from your flashcards, or try teaching someone the material to solidify it in your mind.

Step 4: Create Your Environment

It's important to avoid distractions while you study. This includes both the obvious distractions like visitors and the subtle distractions like an uncomfortable chair (or a too-comfortable couch that makes you want to fall asleep). Set up the best study environment possible: good lighting and a comfortable work area. If background music helps you focus, you may want to turn it on, but otherwise keep the room quiet. If you are using a computer to take notes, be sure you don't have any other windows open, especially applications like social media, games, or anything else that could distract you. Silence your phone and turn off notifications. Be sure to keep water close by so you stay hydrated while you study (but avoid unhealthy drinks and snacks).

Also, take into account the best time of day to study. Are you freshest first thing in the morning? Try to set aside some time then to work through the material. Is your mind clearer in the afternoon or evening? Schedule your study session then. Another method is to study at the same time of day that

Copyright © Mometrix Media. You have been licensed one copy of this document for personal use only. Any other reproduction or redistribution is strictly prohibited. All rights reserved.
This content is provided for test preparation purposes only and does not imply an endorsement by Mometrix of any particular political, scientific, or religious point of view.

you will take the test, so that your brain gets used to working on the material at that time and will be ready to focus at test time.

Step 5: Study!

Once you have done all the study preparation, it's time to settle into the actual studying. Sit down, take a few moments to settle your mind so you can focus, and begin to follow your study plan. Don't give in to distractions or let yourself procrastinate. This is your time to prepare so you'll be ready to fearlessly approach the test. Make the most of the time and stay focused.

Of course, you don't want to burn out. If you study too long you may find that you're not retaining the information very well. Take regular study breaks. For example, taking five minutes out of every hour to walk briskly, breathing deeply and swinging your arms, can help your mind stay fresh.

As you get to the end of each chapter or section, it's a good idea to do a quick review. Remind yourself of what you learned and work on any difficult parts. When you feel that you've mastered the material, move on to the next part. At the end of your study session, briefly skim through your notes again.

But while review is helpful, cramming last minute is NOT. If at all possible, work ahead so that you won't need to fit all your study into the last day. Cramming overloads your brain with more information than it can process and retain, and your tired mind may struggle to recall even previously learned information when it is overwhelmed with last-minute study. Also, the urgent nature of cramming and the stress placed on your brain contribute to anxiety. You'll be more likely to go to the test feeling unprepared and having trouble thinking clearly.

So don't cram, and don't stay up late before the test, even just to review your notes at a leisurely pace. Your brain needs rest more than it needs to go over the information again. In fact, plan to finish your studies by noon or early afternoon the day before the test. Give your brain the rest of the day to relax or focus on other things, and get a good night's sleep. Then you will be fresh for the test and better able to recall what you've studied.

Step 6: Take a practice test

Many courses offer sample tests, either online or in the study materials. This is an excellent resource to check whether you have mastered the material, as well as to prepare for the test format and environment.

Check the test format ahead of time: the number of questions, the type (multiple choice, free response, etc.), and the time limit. Then create a plan for working through them. For example, if you have 30 minutes to take a 60-question test, your limit is 30 seconds per question. Spend less time on the questions you know well so that you can take more time on the difficult ones.

If you have time to take several practice tests, take the first one open book, with no time limit. Work through the questions at your own pace and make sure you fully understand them. Gradually work up to taking a test under test conditions: sit at a desk with all study materials put away and set a timer. Pace yourself to make sure you finish the test with time to spare and go back to check your answers if you have time.

After each test, check your answers. On the questions you missed, be sure you understand why you missed them. Did you misread the question (tests can use tricky wording)? Did you forget the information? Or was it something you hadn't learned? Go back and study any shaky areas that the practice tests reveal.

Copyright © Mometrix Media. You have been licensed one copy of this document for personal use only. Any other reproduction or redistribution is strictly prohibited. All rights reserved.
This content is provided for test preparation purposes only and does not imply an endorsement by Mometrix of any particular political, scientific, or religious point of view.

Taking these tests not only helps with your grade, but also aids in combating test anxiety. If you're already used to the test conditions, you're less likely to worry about it, and working through tests until you're scoring well gives you a confidence boost. Go through the practice tests until you feel comfortable, and then you can go into the test knowing that you're ready for it.

Test Tips

On test day, you should be confident, knowing that you've prepared well and are ready to answer the questions. But aside from preparation, there are several test day strategies you can employ to maximize your performance.

First, as stated before, get a good night's sleep the night before the test (and for several nights before that, if possible). Go into the test with a fresh, alert mind rather than staying up late to study.

Try not to change too much about your normal routine on the day of the test. It's important to eat a nutritious breakfast, but if you normally don't eat breakfast at all, consider eating just a protein bar. If you're a coffee drinker, go ahead and have your normal coffee. Just make sure you time it so that the caffeine doesn't wear off right in the middle of your test. Avoid sugary beverages, and drink enough water to stay hydrated but not so much that you need a restroom break 10 minutes into the test. If your test isn't first thing in the morning, consider going for a walk or doing a light workout before the test to get your blood flowing.

Allow yourself enough time to get ready, and leave for the test with plenty of time to spare so you won't have the anxiety of scrambling to arrive in time. Another reason to be early is to select a good seat. It's helpful to sit away from doors and windows, which can be distracting. Find a good seat, get out your supplies, and settle your mind before the test begins.

When the test begins, start by going over the instructions carefully, even if you already know what to expect. Make sure you avoid any careless mistakes by following the directions.

Then begin working through the questions, pacing yourself as you've practiced. If you're not sure on an answer, don't spend too much time on it, and don't let it shake your confidence. Either skip it and come back later, or eliminate as many wrong answers as possible and guess among the remaining ones. Don't dwell on these questions as you continue—put them out of your mind and focus on what lies ahead.

Be sure to read all of the answer choices, even if you're sure the first one is the right answer. Sometimes you'll find a better one if you keep reading. But don't second-guess yourself if you do immediately know the answer. Your gut instinct is usually right. Don't let test anxiety rob you of the information you know.

If you have time at the end of the test (and if the test format allows), go back and review your answers. Be cautious about changing any, since your first instinct tends to be correct, but make sure you didn't misread any of the questions or accidentally mark the wrong answer choice. Look over any you skipped and make an educated guess.

At the end, leave the test feeling confident. You've done your best, so don't waste time worrying about your performance or wishing you could change anything. Instead, celebrate the successful

Copyright © Mometrix Media. You have been licensed one copy of this document for personal use only. Any other reproduction or redistribution is strictly prohibited. All rights reserved.
This content is provided for test preparation purposes only and does not imply an endorsement by Mometrix of any particular political, scientific, or religious point of view.

completion of this test. And finally, use this test to learn how to deal with anxiety even better next time.

Review Video: 5 Tips to Beat Test Anxiety
Visit mometrix.com/academy and enter code: 570656

Important Qualification

Not all anxiety is created equal. If your test anxiety is causing major issues in your life beyond the classroom or testing center, or if you are experiencing troubling physical symptoms related to your anxiety, it may be a sign of a serious physiological or psychological condition. If this sounds like your situation, we strongly encourage you to seek professional help.

Copyright © Mometrix Media. You have been licensed one copy of this document for personal use only. Any other reproduction or redistribution is strictly prohibited. All rights reserved.
This content is provided for test preparation purposes only and does not imply an endorsement by Mometrix of any particular political, scientific, or religious point of view.

Thank You

We at Mometrix would like to extend our heartfelt thanks to you, our friend and patron, for allowing us to play a part in your journey. It is a privilege to serve people from all walks of life who are unified in their commitment to building the best future they can for themselves.

The preparation you devote to these important testing milestones may be the most valuable educational opportunity you have for making a real difference in your life. We encourage you to put your heart into it—that feeling of succeeding, overcoming, and yes, conquering will be well worth the hours you've invested.

We want to hear your story, your struggles and your successes, and if you see any opportunities for us to improve our materials so we can help others even more effectively in the future, please share that with us as well. **The team at Mometrix would be absolutely thrilled to hear from you!** So please, send us an email (support@mometrix.com) and let's stay in touch.

If you'd like some additional help, check out these other resources we offer for your exam:
http://mometrixflashcards.com/ARRT

Copyright © Mometrix Media. You have been licensed one copy of this document for personal use only. Any other reproduction or redistribution is strictly prohibited. All rights reserved.
This content is provided for test preparation purposes only and does not imply an endorsement by Mometrix of any particular political, scientific, or religious point of view.

Additional Bonus Material

Due to our efforts to try to keep this book to a manageable length, we've created a link that will give you access to all of your additional bonus material:

mometrix.com/bonus948/vascsono

Copyright © Mometrix Media. You have been licensed one copy of this document for personal use only. Any other reproduction or redistribution is strictly prohibited. All rights reserved.
This content is provided for test preparation purposes only and does not imply an endorsement by Mometrix of any particular political, scientific, or religious point of view.